How to integrate water, sanitation and hygiene into HIV programmes

"We shall not finally defeat AIDS, tuberculosis, malaria, or any other infectious diseases that plague the developing world until we have won the battle for safe drinking water, sanitation and basic health care"

Kofi Annan, former UN Secretary-General

WHO Library Cataloguing-in-Publication Data:
How to integrate water, sanitation and hygiene into HIV Programmes.

1.Sanitation – standards. 2.Water quality. 3.Hygiene – standards. 4.Water supply – standards. 5.HIV infections – prevention and control. 6.National health programs. 7.Public policy. I.World Health Organization.

ISBN 978 92 4 154801 4   (NLM Classification: WA 675)

© World Health Organization 2010

Cover designed by Design ONE, Canberra, Australia

Printed in Switzerland

Contents

Tables

Boxes

Foreword

Water, sanitation and hygiene (WASH) practices are essential for maintaining health, yet most countries and donors have not included WASH in national policies and programmes for human immunodeficiency virus (HIV).

The World Health Organization (WHO) and the United States Agency for International Development (USAID) have begun to explore how to integrate WASH into HIV programming. In particular, the United States Centers for Disease Control and Prevention developed and studied approaches to providing safe drinking water for people living with HIV.

Since 2006, WHO and USAID have supported pioneering applications that have integrated WASH into HIV programmes in three countries – Ethiopia, Malawi and Uganda. In addition, USAID has promoted the integration of WASH into different United States Government HIV programmes through various working groups of the President's Emergency Plan for AIDS Response. Many different donors, organizations and programmes are now considering WASH when developing HIV policies and programmes, and are seeking more guidance on how to integrate WASH practices into their programmes. This practical document is a response to such requests.

Our colleagues around the world who have reviewed this document believe that it is a valuable publication. We hope that you will find the document useful in your work to improve the health and lives of people living with HIV.

Merri Weinger	**Yves Chartier**
USAID	WHO
mweinger@usaid.gov	chartiery@who.int
http://www.usaid.gov	http://www.who.int

Acknowledgements

This publication was written by Renuka Bery and Julia Rosenbaum of the Academy for Educational Development (AED), the organization that manages the USAID-funded Hygiene Improvement Project (USAID/HIP). The publication draws on experiences and materials developed by USAID/HIP and others over the past three years. Kate Tulenko of the World Bank, Water and Sanitation Programme wrote the initial water, sanitation and hygiene (WASH) and human immunodeficiency virus (HIV) literature review that was then adapted by the two authors and appears in Annex 2.

Julie Chitty, Public Health Specialist and independent consultant, authored several documents, written for a government audience, which were adapted and included in this publication. WASH–HIV integration training workshops were developed by Eleonore Seumo, AED; Julia Rosenbaum, AED; Elizabeth Younger, Manoff Group; Marie Coughlan, Save the Children/US; and Julie Chitty, USAID/HIP consultant. Again, this material has been adapted into job aids and included as an annex. Lonna Shafritz, AED, provided valuable research efforts and a welcome critical input in relation to structuring the document. Orlando Hernandez, AED, developed the monitoring indicators in collaboration with the authors.

Merri Weinger, USAID and Yves Chartier, World Health Organization (WHO) have championed and supported pioneering WASH–HIV integration activities in three countries; without these activities, we could not have written this document. The communities of practice and country teams that have pioneered WASH–HIV integration include:

- in Malawi, Antonia Powell, Catholic Relief Services (CRS), and her team;

- in Ethiopia, Mesfin Tesfay, AED, and the Water and Sanitation Programme;

- in Uganda, Lucy Korukiiku, AED, and the Plan International team.

Peer review and comments were provided from the following experts: Sandra Callier, AED; Julie Chitty, USAID/HIP consultant; Libertad Gonzalez, International Red Cross and Red Crescent Society; Ben Harvey, International Rescue Committee; Orlando Hernandez, AED; Peter Maes, Médecins Sans Frontières (MSF); Patricia Mantey, AED; Maryline Mulemba, MSF; Alana Potter, International Water and Sanitation Centre, Netherlands; Antonia Powell, CRS; Robert Quick, US Centers for Disease Control and Prevention; Shannon Senefeld, CRS; Foyeke Tolani, Oxfam, UK; Nathalie van Meerbeeck, MSF; Dennis Warner, CRS; and Elizabeth Younger, Manoff Group.

This guideline will be reviewed five years after its publication.

The development of this guideline and the editing were coordinated by Merri Weinger, USAID; Anne Kerisel, WHO consultant; and Yves Chartier, WHO, and was made possible with the support of USAID.

A detailed information on the process development of this guideline is in Annex 1.

This guideline was jointly funded and produced by the United States Agency for International Development and the World Health Organization.

Declarations of interest

The two authors (Renuka Bery and Julia Rosenbaum) signed conflict of interest statements. No conflicts of interest in terms of receiving commercial or non-commercial support were declared by the two authors. The peer reviewers did not declare any conflict of interest. The affiliations of all group members are listed in Annex 1.

Acronyms and abbreviations

AED	Academy for Educational Development
AIDS	acquired immunodeficiency syndrome
ART	antiretroviral therapy
CDC	Centers for Disease Control and Prevention
COP	community of practice
CRS	Catholic Relief Services
HIP	Hygiene Improvement Project
HIV	human immunodeficiency virus
NaDCC	sodium dichloroisocyanurate
NGO	nongovernmental organization
OSSA	Organization for Social Services for AIDS
PEPFAR	President's Emergency Plan for AIDS Relief
PLHIV	people living with HIV
PMTCT	prevention of mother-to-child transmission of HIV
PSI	Population Services International
SODIS	solar disinfection
UN	United Nations
UNICEF	United Nations Children's Fund
US	United States
USAID	United States Agency for International Development
UV	ultraviolet
WASH	water, sanitation and hygiene
WHO	World Health Organization
WSP	Water and Sanitation Programme, World Bank

Executive summary

The term 'WASH' is used to refer to:

- *water* – access to water, and consideration of issues of quantity and quality;

- *sanitation* – safe handling and disposal of human excreta (faeces, urine, menstrual blood, sputum and sweat), management of wastes (including trash, wastewater, storm water, sewage and hazardous wastes) and control of disease vectors (such as mosquitoes and flies);

- *hygiene practices* – in particular, effective hand washing.

WASH practices are essential for maintaining people's health and dignity, and a growing body of literature has demonstrated that WASH practices are particularly important in programmes to reduce the impact of HIV and AIDS. Yet the knowledge and tools that make improved WASH practices possible are beyond the means of many people, especially people living with HIV (PLHIV).

This document is the first comprehensive guide to integrating WASH practices into HIV care. It was written in response to requests from countries and programmes for clear instruction on how to develop care programmes at the national level. It contains guidance on implementing priority WASH practices, including WASH in global and national HIV/AIDS policy and guidance, and integrating WASH–HIV programmes. WASH practices benefit everyone, and integrating WASH into HIV programmes provides additional opportunities and resources to improve public health outcomes for all.

Implementing priority WASH practices

The priority actions to integrate into national HIV programmes are:

- *Treat drinking water* – even where a reliable source of safe water is available, it is often difficult to assure safe transport and storage practices; it is therefore good practice to treat drinking water where it is used, using chlorination systems, solar disinfection, boiling or filtration.

- *Store treated drinking water safely* – ideally, treated water would be stored in a vessel or container with a narrow mouth and lid to prevent recontamination of treated water, and preferably a tap or spigot.

- *Promote hand washing* – programmes should provide guidance and training on washing hands at critical times and with proper technique across all HIV programmes (e.g. home, community, school and facility-based programmes); and place hand-washing stations with needed supplies (soap or ash, and water) in programme sites.

- *Handle and dispose of faeces safely* – programmes should support construction of simple, on-site waste disposal systems such as latrines and, for those clients without bowel control or with mobility problems, promote simple methods to handle and dispose of faeces safely in clinical settings and in households.

- *Manage menstruation* – steps include safe disposal of items soaked in menstrual blood, or cleaning them for re-use.

- *Prepare, handle and store food safely* – sanitary food preparation, handling and storage can prevent diarrhoea; special food hygiene behaviours should be practised when preparing food for infants and young children.

- *Promote personal cleanliness of PLHIV and their environment* – simple steps can prevent the spread of infection, boost client morale and improve the health of HIV-affected communities; these steps include bathing daily with soap, washing clothing and bed linen regularly, and controlling animals.

When implementing the priority WASH practices, the focus should be on measures considered feasible by the householder, taking into account the current practice, the available resources and the particular social context. The home visitor, counsellor, family member or clinician must assess what the current barriers are to each WASH practice, and how they can be overcome. They can then negotiate a commitment to try a few practices that seem feasible, worth changing and safe, from the point of view of the householder.

Including WASH in global and national HIV/AIDS policy and guidance

A systematic review of HIV and AIDS policies and guidelines from 14 countries demonstrated that details of specific wash actions were often lacking. The WASH areas most frequently addressed were safe drinking water and safe food consumption. A few documents mentioned hand washing, faeces disposal and personal hygiene, but this material was often located in the background information. No document mentioned anything about water quantity or storage, menstrual blood management, or adaptation of sanitation and water supply systems for people with mobility restrictions. Also, these documents provided almost no information on how to practise WASH actions.

Steps to integrate WASH into global HIV/AIDS policy and guidance include:

- modifying reference documents used to develop country policies and guidelines;

- revising minimum packages, home-based care kits, school-based HIV education kits, indicator lists and monitoring forms to include WASH;

- ensuring that policies and guidelines suggest environmental health collaboration at all levels, as part of the multisectoral focus;

- learning from other multisectoral interventions;

- developing a list of key WASH behaviours for PLHIV.

On the national level, it is not necessary to develop a free-standing WASH and HIV policy; instead, it is best to integrate WASH policies and guidance into overall HIV policies, whether general HIV or area-specific. Countries can improve WASH guidance when writing or revising HIV-related policies, guidelines and handbooks by including specific details such as water access, water quantity, sanitation, hygiene and hand-washing knowledge and practice.

This document provides examples of specific language that can be used to modify HIV/AIDS policies and related materials.

Integrating WASH–HIV programmes

HIV and AIDS are often characterized as health issues and are therefore not integrated into plans and activities of other sectors. In particular, ministries of health and ministries of water and/or sanitation rarely coordinate or develop joint plans. To integrate HIV and WASH programmes, the sectors should consider protecting human resources through HIV prevention and mitigation programmes, and consider the special hardware needs of those affected by HIV in WASH programmes and activities.

Comprehensive WASH strategies include a wide range of interventions to improve the quality of life for PLHIV and their families. These interventions are not specific to any one setting or location, and are generally delivered through the home, community, school or facility. WASH interventions cannot be standardized for all situations and countries; interventions should be designed to suit local priorities and resources.

This document is the first to systematically bring together information on integrating WASH and HIV to assist country-level programming. It is presented as a step towards the goal of making WASH a routine part of HIV prevention and care, and HIV considerations a routine part of water and sanitation programmes around the world.

1   Introduction

1.1   Overview

Water, sanitation and hygiene are essential for maintaining people's health and dignity. The term 'WASH' is used to refer to:

- *water* – access to water, and consideration of issues of quantity and quality;

- *sanitation* – safe handling and disposal of human excreta (faeces, urine, menstrual blood, sputum and sweat), management of wastes (including trash, wastewater, storm water, sewage and hazardous wastes) and control of disease vectors (such as mosquitoes and flies);

- *hygiene practices* – in particular, effective hand washing.

A small but growing body of literature has demonstrated the importance of WASH in programmes that aim to reduce the impact of HIV (human immunodeficiency virus) and AIDS (acquired immunodeficiency syndrome). People living with HIV (PLHIV) have compromised immune systems, making them more susceptible to opportunistic infections, such as diarrhoea and skin diseases. For example, diarrhoea rates are 2–6 times higher in PLHIV than in those who are not infected, and rates of acute and persistent diarrhoea are twice as high in populations of PLHIV as in uninfected populations (Lule et al., 2005). Infections reduce the quality of life of people living with HIV (PLHIV) and can speed the progression from HIV to AIDS. Diarrhoeal diseases also reduce the absorption of antiretroviral medicines and essential nutrients (Bushen et al., 2004). WASH practices, such as hand washing, sanitation, and water treatment and safe storage have each been proven to reduce diarrhoea rates by 30–40% (Curtis & Cairncross, 2003; Fewtrell et al., 2005; Clasen et al., 2007).

WASH practices also help to prevent caregivers and other household members from contracting water-related diarrhoeal diseases. A healthier and stronger household is more economically viable and resilient in the face of the challenges of HIV.

Despite the clear benefits of WASH practices, meeting the WASH needs of PLHIV is an enormous challenge. The people with the greatest needs are often the most disenfranchised and vulnerable, and often have the fewest resources available to solve problems in sustainable ways. WASH practices benefit everyone, and integrating WASH into HIV programmes provides additional opportunities and resources to improve overall public health outcomes.

1.1.1 Purpose and scope

The benefits of integrating WASH practices into HIV care and support programmes are clear. However, information on how to integrate these practices has only emerged recently, and has not yet been applied to HIV policies and programmes at the national level. This document is the first comprehensive guide to integrating WASH practices into HIV care. It was written in response to requests from countries and programmes for clear instruction on developing care programmes at the national level. The document encourages all WASH and HIV practitioners to work towards integrating WASH practices into HIV care, and to document, share and promote their experiences widely to improve people's lives.

1.1.2 Target audience

This document is mainly aimed at those managing and implementing programmes in national governments; specifically, at directors of HIV care and support programmes, under ministries of health and national AIDS commissions. It also targets those within nongovernmental organizations (NGOs) who manage or implement HIV and AIDS programmes in areas such as prevention of mother-to-child transmission (PMTCT), care and treatment, nutrition, paediatrics, and orphans and vulnerable children. A secondary audience is water and sanitation sector programme planners, who can use this document to start integrating HIV considerations into water and sanitation programming.

1.1.3 Objectives

The objective of this document is to facilitate the integration of WASH into official HIV guidelines and standards, and into HIV programming. The document:

- outlines *why* WASH should be included in HIV programmes;
- details *which* WASH practices to include in HIV programmes;
- identifies *how* WASH can be included in HIV programmes, illustrated by case studies from various countries;
- provides concrete recommendations for country programmes and those implementing them on how to integrate WASH into HIV policies and programmes.

1.1.4 Structure of this document

This chapter provides an overview of the document and some background on the evidence of the importance of WASH, the burden of unsafe water and sanitation, and effective WASH practices.

Chapter 2 provides guidance on the WASH practices that national HIV/AIDS programmes should implement as a priority, and outlines a recommended approach for improving WASH practices. The chapter includes detailed descriptions of recommended practices such as steps for hand washing, strategies for treating water and methods of food handling.

Chapter 3 describes steps to integrate WASH into key HIV-related reference documents such as policies, guidelines and handbooks, on a national and global level.

Chapter 4 provides examples of specific language that can be used to modify HIV/AIDS policies and related materials, using safe drinking water as an example.

Chapter 5 presents interventions that could be considered for programme approaches for WASH–HIV integration, depending on local priorities and resources. The chapter includes practical case studies to provide snapshots of the types of integrated HIV–WASH interventions that different programmes are trying around the world.

The annexes provide practical tools that can be adapted to the local context, and more detailed descriptions of the evidence and literature on WASH and HIV.

1.2 Background

1.2.1 Evidence for the importance of WASH

This section summarizes the evidence for the importance of WASH in relation to HIV, and for what works in reducing rates of opportunistic infections.

Water

Access

Access to safe water is considered a basic human need and, in most countries, a basic human right (Kamminga & Wegelin-Schuringa, 2005). Yet many people in developing countries, especially in rural communities, lack access to safe water. The negative effects of lack of access to sufficient quantities of water, water of reasonable quality, basic sanitation and hygiene are magnified for HIV-infected, immunocompromised individuals. The added burden of unsafe water affects not only PLHIV, but the entire family, increasing the risk of diarrhoeal disease and lost productivity.

Quantity

The World Health Organization (WHO) recommends a minimum of 20 litres of water per person per day, to cover consumption, food preparation, cleaning, laundering and personal hygiene. For a person living with HIV, the needs can increase significantly, to over 100 litres per day, as shown by Table 1.1.

Table 1.1   Basic water needs of people living with HIV and AIDS

Water need	Water required
Basic water for drinking, food preparation, laundering and personal hygiene	20 l per day (recommended minimum)
Water for taking antiretroviral medications	Additional 1.5 l per day
Water for replacement feeding of infants under 6 months	Minimum 1 l per day (without water needed for cleaning)
Water for replacement feeding of infants over 6 months	2 l per day (without water needed for cleaning)
Cleaning PLHIV and laundering clothes and bedding (daily during bouts of diarrhoea)	20–80 l per day[a]
Total	**Approximately 100 l per day**

AIDS, acquired immunodeficiency syndrome; PLHIV, people living with human immunodeficiency virus.
[a] Depending whether or not the patient is under antiretroviral treatment.
Source: Ngwenya & Kgathi, 2006; Molose, Potter & Mvula Trust, 2007; WSP, 2007.

Quality

Piped water is available in some areas, but is often untreated or is contaminated between the source and the home. Simple, low-cost strategies for treating and safely storing water at the household level can greatly improve the microbial quality of water and can reduce diarrhoeal disease by 30–40%, achieving outcomes comparable to those achieved by hand washing and safe handling and disposal of faeces (Sobsey, 2002; USAID, 2004).

Several technologies are viable for treating water in the home; they include chlorination; use of various types of filters; proper boiling (i.e. to a rolling boil); solar disinfection (SODIS) using heat and ultraviolet (UV) radiation; and combined chemical coagulation, flocculation and disinfection. A study in Uganda (Lule et al., 2005) showed that disinfection of water using a simple, home-based system consisting of a chlorine solution followed by storage in a container with a narrow mouth, lid and a spigot, led to a greater than 30% decrease in frequency of diarrhoea in PLHIV and also decreased the severity of diarrhoea. When combined with prophylaxis using a locally available antibiotic (cotrimoxazole), safe treatment and storage of water reduced diarrhoea episodes by 67% in PLHIV.

Sanitation

PLHIV are particularly susceptible to contracting diarrhoea when any faecal matter is present in the environment. More than half of PLHIV suffer from chronic diseases (Curtis & Cairncross, 2003). Safe handling and disposal of faeces can reduce the risk of diarrhoeal disease by 30% or more (Fewtrell et al., 2005). For example, in a recent field trial in Uganda, the presence of a latrine in a compound was associated with fewer episodes of diarrhoea and fewer days of diarrhoea in PLHIV (Lule et al., 2005).

Hygiene

Hand washing

If done properly and at critical times, washing hands with soap or an abrasive substance such as ash is effective in preventing diarrhoea. A meta-analysis of hand-washing studies conducted in developing countries concluded that hand washing can reduce the risk of diarrhoea in the general population by 42–44% (Curtis & Cairncross, 2003). Similarly, a study in Uganda demonstrated that the presence of soap in the house was associated with fewer days with diarrhoea (Lule et al., 2005), inferring that washing hands reduces diarrhoea.

Menstruation management

Hygiene, disease and menstrual blood in HIV-infected women are not discussed in the literature; only the grey (unpublished) literature and anecdotal conversations between scientists and programme managers have covered this topic. Before antiretroviral therapy (ART) became prevalent, women often stopped menstruating once HIV had advanced. However, now that ART is widely used even in resource-poor countries, women continue to menstruate, which poses a hygiene challenge and possible risk of HIV transmission to caregivers. Menstrual blood of HIV-positive women contains the virus, sometimes at a higher load than regular blood (Reichelderfer et al., 2000). Thus, HIV-positive women and their caregivers must prevent HIV transmission from menstrual blood by practising universal precautions.[1]

Food hygiene

Every year, an estimated 1.8 million people die as a result of diarrhoeal diseases; most of these cases can be attributed to contaminated food or water.[2] For example, raw fruits and vegetables, and undercooked or spoiled meat, poultry, fish or eggs are often contaminated with microorganisms that cause diarrhoea (WHO, 2009a). A breastfeeding study in Kisumu, Kenya, illustrated that diarrhoea is not always caused by poor quality water, but can also be caused by unhygienic food and exposure to faeces in the environment (Harris et al., 2009). Whether weaning foods are contaminated depends largely on the food type, storage time, ambient storage temperature, storage method and the temperature reached on re-warming before feeding (Lantana, 2003; WHO, 2010).

---

[1] As defined by the US Centers for Disease Control and Prevention, universal precautions apply to blood, other body fluids containing visible blood, semen and vaginal secretions. Practising universal precautions involves using protective barriers (e.g. gloves, gowns, masks or protective eyewear) to reduce a caregiver's risk of exposure to materials potentially infected with HIV or other bloodborne pathogens.
[2] http://www.who.int/water_sanitation_health/publications/factsfigures04/en

1.2.2 Burden of unsafe water and sanitation

Water and sanitation issues are important to everyone, in whatever context, to keep people safe from diarrhoeal diseases. Water and sanitation issues affect the health of infants and young children, and place a particular burden on women and girls, especially in an HIV context. The key issues are described below. Although they may not be specifically related to HIV, these issues are particularly important in the context of HIV, where preventing diarrhoea in the whole family reduces burdens on caregivers and keeps PLHIV healthier.

Many common infections that cause diarrhoea can spread from one person to another when people defecate in the open air. Intestinal worms, which are transmitted when people ingest faecal matter in unclean water or step in it with bare feet, divert around one third of the food a child consumes, and impair a child's health, nutrition and cognitive development. Malnutrition is a contributing factor to over 50% of childhood illness (UN-Water, 2008).

Women and girls

Water issues affect women and girls differently to men and boys. Across many countries, girls reportedly spend up to three hours each day fetching water and cleaning latrines. Women and girls are the primary caregivers for the chronically ill, and women now compose the majority of PLHIV in many countries.

Infants and young children

Diarrhoea accounts for nearly 20% of child deaths worldwide, largely through unsafe drinking water, inadequate sanitation and poor hygiene (Morris, Black & Tomaskovic, 2003). Although some cultures do not consider infant faeces infectious, when contaminated with pathogens it is as infectious as adult faeces and must be disposed of safely. The youngest children are much more likely than adults to become ill from eating contaminated food or drinking contaminated water.

School children

African countries typically recommend one toilet per 30 students; however, studies conducted by the Rockefeller Foundation have found that some schools have only one toilet per 200 students, or have no toilets at all, let alone hand-washing points. In Nigeria, the national toilet-to-pupil ratio is one latrine to 292 students, but a national target ratio of one latrine to 40 pupils is being pursued (UNICEF & IRC International Water and Sanitation Centre, 2005). Despite the challenges, there are simple, high-impact interventions that can be used to prevent diarrhoea and worm infestation in children. For example, a Kenyan school reduced diarrhoeal episodes in school children by promoting hand washing, and by treating and safely storing drinking water at the point of use, despite the fact that the water source was an unprotected shallow well (O'Reilly et al., 2008). Access to hygienic toilets can reduce child diarrhoeal deaths by more than 30% and prevent some worm infestations in children (UN-Water, 2008). Isolated latrines without lights are often associated with sexual violence towards school children, which carries the potential for HIV transmission.

Although poverty is still a leading factor in determining school attendance, young women attending school have special needs that are now becoming better understood (WHO, 2009b). UNICEF estimates that about 1 in 10 African school-age girls do not attend school during menstruation or drop out when puberty starts, because schools lack clean and private sanitation facilities. Regular absence from school for several days each month can, even in the short term, have a negative impact on a girl's learning and hence on her academic performance. For girls who cannot afford to buy washing soap, it may be difficult to clean uniforms or school clothes regularly, and this may prevent many girls from attending school. However, simple approaches such as adequate gender-specific latrines can ensure that children, especially girls, are not excluded from fully participating in the educational system because of their maturing bodies.

Orphans and vulnerable children

Many children are affected by HIV – either when their parents die or because they are living in households with HIV-infected individuals – and have greater responsibilities or less access to basic needs. Targeting programmes that provide services to orphans and vulnerable children with WASH messages and practices helps to prevent the spread of pathogens that cause diarrhoea, and skin and eye diseases.

Stigma

Stigma against HIV and AIDS is a hidden epidemic that is as large as, or even larger than the HIV epidemic itself. PLHIV face different types of discrimination that affect housing, employment, social interactions, childcare, and access to medical services, water and sanitation (Magrath & Tesfu, 2006).

Although the WASH needs of PLHIV are greater than those without HIV, PLHIV often have less access to water and sanitation facilities than their neighbours because of sickness or discrimination (Magrath & Tesfu, 2006). PLHIV and their families have been subjected to discrimination if a person's HIV status is known; for example, sometimes PLHIV are refused the right to use communal latrines because users fear that HIV can be transmitted through latrines (Magrath & Tesfu, 2006). Therefore, many clients go to distant cities to get their medicines to avoid being recognized at a local health clinic (OSSA/Bahir Dar, personal communication, 2009). Also, in some communities, a person with diarrhoea is considered to be infected with HIV, whether that person's HIV status is known or not.

Special equipment or new technologies that target HIV programmes specifically while addressing real needs of PLHIV can inadvertently contribute to stigma and discrimination. In Ethiopia, some PLHIV learned about using a water-saving hand-washing device called a tippy tap[1] from home-based care workers working for an HIV support organization. Although many clients adopted the tippy tap, other clients said making such a device would identify them to their neighbours as HIV positive (Tesfagoh/Bahir Dar, personal communication, 2009). In Uganda, one programme gave clients a water container with a spigot and a hypochlorite solution to treat their water. Anecdotal evidence indicates that because the water container was not local, everyone in the community knew that people with those water containers were HIV positive.

1.2.3   Effective WASH approaches

It is clear that practical improvements in WASH can improve the lives of people living with HIV/AIDS and their families. However, this area of integration is only now emerging as a programming option, and there are few rigorous programme evaluations to show which programming approaches are most effective. Box 1.1, below, summarizes what is already known.

Over the next few years, relevant and vital field data will emerge on programming techniques, as integration efforts are more systematically evaluated. This information will show which approaches to integrating WASH into HIV programmes are most effective at improving health outcomes.

The remaining chapters of this document provide guidance for making decisions on integration of WASH into HIV programmes. The guidance is based on the evidence and on what can reasonably be inferred from the data.

---

[1] A tippy tap is a simple plastic jug, gourd or local receptacle with a tap or opening that provides a slow, steady stream of water for washing hands with very little water. (See Annex 2: Making a tippy tap.)

Box 1.1   Evidence from programme evaluations

This box summarizes evidence from programme evaluations on effective and cost-effective WASH interventions.

Using a safe water system reduces diarrhoea and death in high HIV incidence areas

A study in western Kenya (in a general population with high HIV rates) noted that 43% fewer deaths occurred using the Safe Water System or PUR (Crump et al., 2005). The study found that the presence of residual chlorine correlated more closely with risk reduction than did a good container. In large, uncovered clay pots, where drinking water is kept for up to three days, chlorine disappears in one day.

Drinking safe water, presence of soap, and presence of a latrine mean fewer and shorter bouts of diarrhoea in PLHIV and their affected families, and fewer missed days of work and school

People who drank water outside the home saw fewer benefits than those who consistently drank treated water. An evaluation of a basic care package in Uganda demonstrated that use of a safe water system must be consistent. In general, there is a high uptake of safe water systems if the distribution is clinic based, whereas community-based promotion shows mixed results (Lule et al., 2005).

Softening food for PLHIV with clean water helps them to ingest food

In advanced stages of AIDS, PLHIV often have mouth sores that make eating difficult. Softening food with water helps PLHIV ingest the food, which is important for maintaining good nutrition (WELL Project, 2004a; Kamminga & Wegelin-Schuringa, 2005).

Focusing on water and sanitation matters, but is not enough

A breastfeeding study conducted by the United States Centers for Disease Control and Prevention (CDC) in Kenya illustrated that diarrhoea is not always caused by poor water, but perhaps also by contaminated food and exposure to faecal pathogens in the environment (Harris et al., 2009).

Addressing WASH needs of PLHIV households can create stigma and discrimination

WASH inputs that target PLHIV households directly can create stigma. Organizations are now designing special WASH considerations to benefit the entire community; for example, considering alternative latrine designs to accommodate weaker individuals who may need assistance (e.g. the less mobile, the disabled, the elderly, children and PLHIV). The NGO WaterAid now discusses water and sanitation needs in terms of inclusiveness, because people with lower social status – whether disabled, PLHIV, elderly or women – often have increased needs but decreased access (Magrath &Tesfu, 2006). Inclusive design means offering a range of options, exploring cost implications and considering everyone's needs rather than targeting a specific audience.

> **Focusing on WASH as part of HIV programmes is cost effective**
>
> A reanalysis (Mermin et al., 2005) of the cost data from the much quoted safe water study in Uganda (Lule et al., 2005) estimated that WASH interventions would cost about the same as the widely accepted and cost-effective expanded programme on immunization (tuberculosis, diphtheria, pertussis, tetanus, polio and measles). By comparison, the cost of ART therapy in Africa is almost 400 times this amount (see Annex 2).

Table 1.2 describes how specific WASH activities can reduce diarrhoea, respiratory illnesses, and skin and eye diseases through different care and treatment programmes.

Table 1.2   WASH actions that support different HIV programmes

Focus of programme	WASH action
Prevention of mother-to-child transmission of HIV	• Use safe water, sanitation and hygiene practices during delivery. • Ensure safe infant feeding: use treated water for replacement feeding and complementary feeding; wash hands with soap before preparing food or feeding. • Wash hands with soap to prepare food and to clean utensils.
Adult care and treatment	• Treat and safely store water for drinking. • Wash hands with soap. • Promote hygienic latrines and labour-saving water and sanitation technologies, or modifications for those with impaired mobility. • Improve personal and environmental cleanliness.
Paediatric care and treatment	• Use treated water for drinking, feeding and safe reconstitution of medicines. • Wash hands with soap. • Safely handle and dispose of children's diapers and faeces; promote a hygienic potty or latrine, etc.
Nutritional care and support	• Use treated water for drinking, food preparation and taking medicines. • Wash hands with soap. • Prepare food safely.
Orphans and vulnerable children	• Treat and safely store drinking water for children in the household. • Wash hands with soap. • Promote hygienic latrine use. • Prepare food safely.

Counselling and testing	• Counsel clients to:
	  – wash hands with soap
	  – treat and safely store drinking water
	  – use a latrine and safely dispose of faeces
	  – wash surfaces used to prepare and eat foods
	  – improve personal and environmental cleanliness.

2 Priority WASH practices to integrate into national HIV/AIDS programmes

This chapter provides guidance on the WASH practices that national HIV/AIDS programmes should implement as a priority. In summary, the practices are to:

- treat drinking water (Section 2.1)
- store treated drinking water safely (Section 2.2)
- promote hand washing (Section 2.3)
- handle and dispose of faeces safely (Section 2.4)
- manage menstruation (Section 2.5)
- prepare, handle and store food safely (Section 2.6)
- promote personal cleanliness of PLHIV and their environment (Section 2.7).

Section 2.8 outlines a recommended approach for improving WASH practices.

2.1 Treat drinking water

Water programmes should provide potable water (e.g. chlorinated piped water, or water from a covered well that is equipped with a hand pump) and help to ensure that transport and storage practices are safe. However, even where a reliable source of safe water is available, it is often difficult to assure safe transport and storage practices. Thus, HIV programmes should support the treatment of drinking water at the point of use (WHO, 2007a) for those who are HIV infected, and promote the safe storage practices listed in section 2.2.

Use of household bleach (sodium hypochlorite) can be effective in treating drinking water, but it is difficult to recommend an effective dose because the bleach concentration varies both within and across brands. A further difficulty is lack of a commonly available standard measure to use as the dosage measurement. There are four main strategies for treating water:

- use a chlorine-releasing compound (this is the most effective strategy, because the chlorine residual lasts for several days);
- use solar disinfection;
- boil water;
- filter water.

Whatever method is used, the treated water should be stored in an appropriate vessel.

2.1.1 Chlorination systems

Apart from boiling, chlorination is the most widely practised means of water treatment at community level. Chlorine treats water for up to seven days if the water is stored in a tightly closed container and no contamination occurs. If drinking water is not in an enclosed storage container, it should be re-treated after 24 hours. The chlorine source can be a bleaching solution (sodium hypochlorite), a bleaching powder (chlorinated lime), calcium hypochlorite or sodium dichloroisocyanurate (NaDCC) tablets, which are usually available and affordable.

When the turbidity of the (raw) water is high, chlorination is not effective. The recommended turbidity value for effective chlorination is set at 5 nephelometric turbidity units (NTU), although turbidities up to 20 NTU can be acceptable for chlorination of water in an acute situation (WHO, 2006, 2008). If this turbidity is exceeded, the turbidity in the raw water has to be reduced. Three options for reducing turbidity, each of which has a proven health impact, are use of:

- a safe water system
- a flocculant or disinfectant powder
- NaDCC tablets.

Safe water system

The safe water system procedure supported by the CDC involves three steps: chlorine treatment (using sodium hypochlorite), a safe storage container with a spigot and behaviour-change techniques. Sodium hypochlorite disinfectant is easy to use and disseminate, although it may have a residual taste and smell. To increase user acceptability, turbid water can first be filtered through a cloth. The safe water system includes an improved storage vessel or container with a narrow mouth, a lid and a tap to prevent recontamination. If such storage vessels are not available locally, two alternatives are a jerry can with a lid or a tightly covered bucket. The most important barrier to infection in this system is the chlorine residual.

Flocculant–disinfectant powder

An example of a flocculant–disinfectant powder is PUR Purifier of Water which contains powdered ferric sulfate (a flocculant) and calcium hypochlorite (a disinfectant). Such powders are particularly effective in removing most bacteria, viruses and protozoa from turbid water; for example, from water drawn from a muddy stream. Using a flocculant–disinfectant powder involves a multistep process.

- Powder is added to an open bucket containing 10 litres of water.

- The water is stirred for 5 minutes.

- The solid particles settle to the bottom of the bucket.

- The water is strained through a cotton cloth into a second container.

- After 20 minutes, depending on the presence of free residual chlorine, the water is safe for drinking.

This product is more expensive than the safe water system and requires more steps (and training and supervision) to treat water. However, it effectively clarifies murky water and removes heavy contaminants. The Red Cross recommends using this product only when water is muddy and other methods are not available. Treated water should be properly stored, as described in section 2.2.

NaDCC tablets

NaDCC tablets are an alternate chlorine source for use in the safe water system. Compared to the chlorine solution, the tablets have benefits such as a long shelf life, resistance to degradation from sunlight, single-use packaging and ease of distribution (due to low weight). Initially used mainly in emergencies, NaDCC is increasingly being used for routine drinking water treatment in urban areas. Treated water should be properly stored, as described in section 2.2.

2.1.2   Solar disinfection

SODIS is practised in 20 countries and uses UV-A radiation from the sun to treat water. The method does not affect the colour, taste, or odour of the water, but it can only be used when the water is clear. SODIS requires transparent, 1–2 litre plastic bottles and a long period of time for effective treatment (six hours in bright sun or two days in cloudy weather). Treating large quantities of water is difficult, because acquiring sufficient plastic bottles is challenging in some locations, treatment is not effective in turbid water and the warm temperature of the water can be a deterrent to consumers. Treated water should be properly stored, as described in section 2.2.

2.1.3   Boiling

WHO and the CDC recommend bringing water to a rolling boil (the point where large bubbles begin to come to the top) to kill pathogens. Boiling has a number of disadvantages, in that it:

- is costly;

- typically requires biomass fuels that can contribute to climate change and deforestation;

- can put small children at risk of burns;

- produces water that is easily recontaminated;

- influences the taste of the water (this can be remedied by re-oxidizing the water by stirring).

Boiled water should be properly stored, as described in section 2.2.

2.1.4 Filtration

Several different filtration methods can be used to treat water for drinking. The ceramic filter is a proven method that reduces microbiological content and decreases diarrhoea. Most ceramic filter systems for treating and storing household water are based on a filter and receptacle model. To use the ceramic filters, the top receptacle (or the ceramic filter itself) is filled with water, which flows through one or more ceramic filters into a storage receptacle. The BioSand Filter – a slow sand filter adapted for use in the home – is widely used. It has been shown to reduce the risk of diarrhoea even though it does not disinfect water as thoroughly as some other technologies. Treated water should be properly stored, as described in section 2.2.

2.2 Store treated drinking water safely

Safe storage of water is critical (WHO, 2007a). Water should be stored in a vessel or container with a narrow mouth and lid to prevent recontamination of treated water, and preferably a tap (although this is often not feasible). If such a vessel is not available, alternatives such as dippers can be substituted for the tap.

- *Ideal option* – The ideal is to store treated water in a vessel or container with a narrow mouth and lid to prevent recontamination of treated water, and preferably with a tap or spigot.

- *Acceptable options* – If the ideal is not available, it is acceptable to:

  - store water in a container with a narrow neck, a jerry can with a lid or a bucket with a tightly fitting lid; and

  - either pour water from the container or use a clean ladle to serve the water.

Whatever type of container is used, it is important to keep hands away from the mouth of the container and to store the container on a shelf away from babies and animals.

Box 2.1 discusses issues in encouraging proper water treatment and storage practices.

> **Box 2.1   Encouraging proper water treatment and storage practices**
>
> Programmes should encourage proper water treatment and storage practices by considering affordability and ease of use. They should also ensure timely replenishment of water-treatment products to avoid running out of stock, which leads to opportunities for contamination. HIV programmes should consider linking with the water sector to improve the number of safe water supply points that are accessible and located near to where they are needed.
>
> Reducing stigma must always be a consideration when promoting new WASH actions. Locally available materials and products should be used wherever possible so that PLHIV are not immediately recognized because they are using a particular technology or apparatus that is not common in the area.

2.3   Promote hand washing

Given the overwhelming evidence in support of hand-washing behaviours, HIV programmes should (WHO, 2009c):

- provide guidance and training on washing hands at critical times and with proper technique across all HIV programmes (e.g. home, community, school and facility-based programmes);
- place hand-washing stations with needed supplies (soap or ash, and water) in programme sites.

2.3.1   Guidance and training on hand washing

Programmes should prioritize washing hands with soap (or ash) at five critical times:

- after defecation
- before preparing food
- before eating food, breastfeeding, or feeding children or PLHIV
- after cleaning up faeces from a child or PLHIV
- before and after caring for patients (WHO, 2009c).

Programmes should encourage a proper hand-washing technique, using the following steps:

1. Wet hands under running water.
2. Rub hands together with soap (or a soap substitute, such as ash).
3. Rinse hands under running (or poured) water.

4. Dry hands thoroughly by shaking them in the air. Towels are not recommended because they are often contaminated, but under certain conditions, programmes could suggest that people dry their hands with a clean, dry towel (preferably a paper towel).

2.3.2　Hand-washing stations and supplies

Hand-washing stations should be placed in health-care facilities (WHO, 2009c), community care points, schools and households to improve hand-washing practice. If possible, the hand-washing station should be conveniently close to where the washing needs to take place (e.g. by the bedside, at the cooking site or near latrines). The stations facilitate hand washing and serve as a reminder to wash hands. Programmes in water-scarce situations or without running water should consider using a tippy tap. Other alternatives for washing hands when no running water is available include a bucket with a tap, or a bucket and pitcher.

2.4　Handle and dispose of faeces safely

Typically, HIV/AIDS programmes have not included construction of simple, on-site waste disposal systems such as latrines. Also, programmes have not supported simple methods to handle and dispose of faeces safely in clinical settings and in households to benefit PLHIV and their families. This section discusses interventions that programmes can introduce to keep clients clean and reduce faeces in the environment. It contains sections for dealing with clients who:

- have bowel control and are mobile

- have bowel control but have problems with mobility

- are bedbound

- lack bowel control.

HIV is apparently not transmitted through blood in faeces; however, many other pathogens are present and it is good practice to use gloves or plastic bags to avoid direct contact with faeces or spreading illnesses. Although this is the ideal, it is rarely feasible in a resource-poor setting. Similarly, the guidance below suggests using gloves or plastic bags, but again this may not be possible in some settings.

2.4.1 Clients with bowel control and mobility

For clients who have bowel control and are mobile, apply the actions listed below.

- *Upgrade existing pit latrines* – Upgrade to meet minimum standards; these include a washable sanitation platform and a cover to the pit. (See Annex 3: Minimum standards ladder diagram.)

- *Clear the path to the latrine* – Remove obstacles such as stones and branches, and fill holes in path.

- *Sensitize and train people in latrine hygiene* – Sensitize people on the need to maintain existing latrines hygienically and train them in how to do so. Priority strategies include promoting latrine cleanliness, use, maintenance and deodorization. Ensure that a latrine is always free of faeces on the platform, seat or other surfaces. No special cleaning is needed after PLHIV use the latrine. A scoop of ash or lime after defecation helps to reduce odour and deter flies.

- *Look at options for accessing a latrine* – If a latrine is not available, consider options for sharing a latrine with others in the community. Leverage support from donors, NGOs and local government to build a latrine or ensure adequate access to one. In the interim, collect and bury or dispose of faeces away from the facility, clinic or home, and away from any area where animals can dig it up.

2.4.2 Clients with bowel control but mobility problems

For clients who have bowel control but have problems with mobility, apply the actions listed below.

- *Install assistive devices if necessary* – If a client is too weak to walk unassisted to an existing latrine, install assistive devices (e.g. poles, ropes or stools) inside or outside the latrine to help a person to reach and use the latrine. (See Annex 3: Latrine designs.)

- *Ensure access to a locally available, simple bedside commode or bedpan* – Provide a commode, bedpan (made of plastic or locally available materials) or squat pot that PLHIV can use to defecate in the bed or house, and that caregivers can empty. Where these items are not accessible, programmes can use locally available materials to create commodes and bedpans. Such materials include buckets, plastic bowls or jerry cans cut in half, gourds, ceramic pots, modified chairs and stools, or any other materials suitable for secure collection of faeces.

- *Encourage proper use and cleaning of a bedside commode or bedpan* – To ensure that a commode or bedpan is used and cleaned properly:

    a. Put a handful of ash or sand in the commode or bedpan before use to prevent solids from sticking.

b. Wipe any faeces from the client's bottom with a disposable cloth or paper; wipe front to back and put the soiled cloth or paper into the commode or bedpan.

c. Place a handful of ash on top of the solids to prevent odours.

d. Dispose of the faeces into a latrine or bury it.

e. Wipe the commode or bedpan to remove any remaining faeces and dispose of the soiled cloth or paper, either putting it into the latrine or burying it, as appropriate.

f. Pour water and bleach solution (9 parts water to 1 part bleach) into the commode or bedpan and leave it for about 20 minutes (WHO, 2007a, 2009b).

g. Empty the bleach solution into a hole (not the latrine) and let the commode or bedpan air dry, in the sun if possible.

h. Wash hands with soap and water. (See Annex 3: Bedpan/commode designs.)

- *Protect the skin, clothing, sheets and mattress of PLHIV and children from becoming soiled with faeces* – Protecting skin, clothing and bedding from soiling helps to reduce the risk that diarrhoea-causing pathogens may spread to other household members and to prevent skin rashes, bed sores and infection. Strategies such as placing a plastic sheet covered by paper or a cloth under the client's buttocks are very simple and cost-effective measures that can ease the caregiving burden. (See Annex 3: Turning bedbound client in bed.)

- *Wash soiled clothes and bed linen* – To wash soiled clothes and linen, first soak the items for 20 minutes in soapy water, then wash them with soap and water, and finally, dry them in the sun. (See Annex 3: Washing clothes and bed linen.)

- *Avoid stigma* – If PLHIV are treated differently from other community or household members and are barred from using a latrine, conduct antistigma and educational opportunities for people to understand that faeces itself does not spread HIV. (See Annex 4 for antistigma activities and references.) The faeces of people with end-stage AIDS are likely to have increased amounts of blood and white blood cells carrying the HIV virus and other infections that could affect household members. As far as possible, caregivers should use gloves or plastic bags to protect their hands when handling faeces.

- *Wash hands after defecation* – Wash hands as specified in section 2.3.1, above. (See Annex 3: Hand washing instructions.)

2.4.3 Clients who are bedbound

For clients who are bedbound, apply the actions listed below.

- *Encourage proper use and cleaning of a bedpan* – For proper use of a bedpan, follow the guidance given in section 2.4.2 (above) for commodes and bedpans, but place the bedpan under the client's buttocks as the person is bedbound.

- *Handle faeces and soiled items hygienically* – Use available materials (e.g. linen, diapers [nappies] or leaves) to assist in hygienic handling of faeces or items soiled with faeces. Use gloves if available; alternatively, use plastic bags to hold soiled linen and faeces.

- *Safely dispose of non-reusable materials* – Where non-reusable materials have been used for cleansing faeces, dispose of them safely; for example, by burning or burying them, or discarding them into a pit latrine.

- *Wash hands after handling faeces or soiled linen* – Wash hands as specified in section 2.3.1, above. (See Annex 3: Hand washing instructions.)

2.4.4 Clients (including children) lacking bowel control

For clients or children who lack bowel control, apply the actions listed below.

- *Use and safely dispose of diapers, or clean rags properly* – Follow steps in Section 2.4.3 to safely dispose of faeces and steps in Section 2.4.2 to safely wash soiled clothes or linen.

- *Ensure safety for children* – Provide small children with potties or partially cover the latrine hole with a small board so children will not fall in.

2.5 Manage menstruation

Any items soaked with menstrual blood – sanitary pads, towels, rags, banana fibres or cloth – must be disposed of appropriately. Soiled materials that will be reused must be cleaned using the process described below. Blood-soaked materials that cannot be reused must be completely burned or discarded in a pit latrine.

Necessary steps for managing menstruation are listed below.

- Soak up blood with sanitary pads, rags or other local materials used.

- Do not store soiled rags for more than a couple of hours. Bloody rags will start to smell, and will attract insects and flies.

- If a woman is bedbound, keep clean rags, washing water and a container for soiled rags near the bed.

- Always protect the hands with gloves or plastic bags when touching someone else's blood, and always wash hands with soap or ash after handling or disposing of materials contaminated with menstrual blood to prevent virus transmission; this is critical even when gloves or bags are used.

- Dispose of blood-soaked materials that cannot be reused (sanitary pads, banana fibres, etc.) in a pit latrine or a shared latrine, or burn these materials completely.

- Wash soiled rags using the following process:

  a) Wash with water and soap, then rinse with water.

  b) Make a dilute bleach solution (9 parts cold water [to prevent stains] to 1 part bleach) and leave blood-soaked rags in this solution for 20 minutes (WHO, 2007a, 2009b).

  c) If no bleach solution is available, soak the rags in soapy water for 20 minutes.

  d) Rinse with soap and water, then again with water only.

  e) Hang rags in the sun to dry.

  f) Keep rags in a dry place for future use.

2.6 Prepare, handle and store food safely

Sanitary food preparation, handling and storage can prevent diarrhoea. This section lists recommendations adapted from guidance provided by the WHO (WHO, 2009a, 2010). These recommendations describe optimal practices, but they may not be feasible in resource-poor contexts. Local adaptations that consider local context and feasibility should be developed and incorporated into national guidance.

The recommendations are listed below.

- *Keep food areas and utensils clean* – Clean all surfaces and equipment used for food preparation with water and soap. Wash utensils with soap (or ash) and water. Protect kitchen areas and food from insects, pests and animals. Use closed containers to keep food protected.

- *Wash hands* – Wash hands as specified in section 2.3.1, above. (See Annex 3: Hand washing instructions.)

- *Separate raw and cooked food* – Keep raw and cooked food separate, to avoid cross contamination. Also:

  – keep equipment and utensils used for handling raw foods separate from those used for cooked foods;

- store cooked foods in proper containers to prevent contact with raw foods;

- use separate plates for raw and cooked foods.

- *Cook food thoroughly* – Bring foods such as soups and stews to a boil to prevent worm infestation.

- *Keep food at safe temperatures* – Do not eat food that has been sitting at room temperature for more than 2 hours. If thawing frozen food, do so in the refrigerator rather than at room temperature. For food that is eaten hot, keep it "piping" hot (i.e. with visible steam rising from it) until served.

- *Use safe water* – Use water that has been treated to make it safe (see section 2.1) to wash raw food, mix with food, make drinks and prepare ice.

- *Practise special food hygiene behaviours for infants and young children* – Infants and young children are particularly susceptible to diarrhoea from unsafe water, food preparation or food storage. Section 2.6.1, below, gives details of special food hygiene behaviours for this age group.

2.6.1 Special food hygiene behaviours for infants and young children

Infants under six months

If a mother or caregiver is unable to practice exclusive breastfeeding for infants under six months, she must follow the WHO's safe infant feeding criteria (Ma et al., 2009; WHO, 2010):[1]

- use a reliable supply of treated water that is stored properly to prepare replacement foods;

- wash hands and utensils thoroughly with soap or ash;

- boil water to prepare foods;

- store unprepared foods in clean, covered containers;

- treat or boil utensils regularly to sterilize them (if boiling is not feasible, use detergent with water treated with chlorine, as this will safely disinfect containers and utensils).

Utensils include feeding bottles, teats, cups and spoons. Keeping bottles and teats clean may be especially difficult in developing country settings, and their use is discouraged. Using a cup and spoon for feeding infants is recommended.

---

[1] In accordance with *How to prepare powdered infant formula in care settings* (WHO and FAO 2007), http://www.fao.org/ag/agn/agns/files/PIF_Care_en.pdf.

Discard prepared feeds, including infant formula, within one hour if the child does not finish the entire portion. Following these precautions can be difficult, but is critical in preventing diarrhoea in young children.

Infants six months and over

Once children reach six months of age, mothers should combine breastfeeding or safe replacement feeding with additional complementary foods. Preparation of such foods requires the same critical hygiene strategies as stated above (i.e. safe water, safe food preparation and safe storage), while the mother and baby continue to be regularly monitored for adequate nutrition. HIV-infected mothers should receive specific counselling and support for at least the first year of the child's life, to ensure adequate infant feeding (WHO, 2010).

Adaptations for resource-poor households

For resource-poor households, the recommendations may be adapted as described below.

- Dedicate a small surface that is easy to clean for food preparation; if possible, this area should be out of reach of small children.

- Create another place to store cleaned dishware. Basic dish racks or tables off the ground will help to avoid utensils coming into contact with soil or animals. If possible, cover this place with a washable surface, such as plastic or a sheet of paper that is changed regularly.

- Clean food preparation surfaces before use with soap and water.

- Cover all raw and cooked foods with a clean cover (e.g. a bowl, plate or plastic film) to keep flies away from the food.

- Heat all food until steam is seen rising from the food.

- Serve food hot.

- Do not eat food that has been sitting at room temperature for more than two hours.

- Treat or boil water used to wash food, mix with food that will not be boiled, make drinks, etc.

2.7   Ensure personal cleanliness of PLHIV and the surrounding environment

The cleanliness of PLHIV, their families, health-care workers and the environment is important in preventing the spread of infection, boosting client morale and achieving a positive health impact for HIV-affected communities. Priority recommendations are listed below.

- *Bathe daily with soap* – When bathing a client, pay special attention to cleaning the person's hands, face, armpits, genital area and anus. Females should always cleanse their genital and anal region from "front-to-back" to avoid contamination. Uncircumcised males should gently pull back the foreskin and clean from the tip of the penis to the shaft. If clients are immobile, they may be bathed in a bed or chair. If a client has a skin condition that worsens with daily baths, adjust the bathing schedule accordingly.

- *Avoid spreading infection through bodily fluids and secretions.*

  - Clean equipment and dressings used in care appropriately.

  - Avoid contact with bodily fluids and secretions, such as the client's urine, vomit or sputum. If possible, cover hands by wearing gloves (or use plastic bags if gloves are not available). Use gloves to protect against bloodborne pathogens.

  - To safely dispose of bodily fluids and secretions, remove spills with a disposable cloth or paper, and then use a dilute bleach solution (9 parts water, 1 part bleach) to decontaminate the soiled area.

- *Wash clothing and bed linen regularly* – See section 2.4.2 (above) for guidance on washing clothing and linen.

- *Remove dirt from surfaces* – Remove dirt by sweeping and dusting, and reduce pathogens by washing with hot soapy water, rinsing, air drying (in direct sunlight if possible), or cleaning with household bleach or other household disinfectant products.

- *Dispose of contaminated material safely* – Place garbage and non-reusable materials that may be contaminated into a waste receptacle, protected pit or latrine.

- *Disinfect key surfaces* – Clean latrines, baths, basins, kitchens, then disinfect using a dilute bleach solution (9 parts water, 1 part bleach) if available; if bleach is not available, clean the surfaces with soap and water.

- *Control animals* – Keep animals away from households, health-care facilities, and food or water sources because they may expose household members to diarrhoeal disease and worm infestation. Control vectors such as flies, mosquitoes, cockroaches and rats by keeping food covered, disposing of faeces properly, and removing or covering standing water and garbage. If necessary, plug holes in walls, and use nets, traps and baits to control pests.

2.8 A recommended approach to improvement of WASH practices

PLHIV, their families, outreach workers and clinicians are not currently practising all the recommended WASH behaviours consistently or correctly. Thus, reducing diarrhoea and improving the quality of life for PLHIV and their families means changing hygiene and sanitation behaviours in all these groups. This document outlines specific WASH behaviours or practices that can be incorporated into guides and programmes.

People's WASH behaviours are based on many different factors, not just their knowledge, attitudes and beliefs. Too often, health promotion efforts focus on educating target audiences, assuming that increased knowledge is the most important factor in encouraging a particular behaviour. For WASH practices, knowledge is essential, but is not sufficient to improve behaviour. Table 2.1 shows some of the other factors that influence behaviour, illustrated by the example of promotion of hand washing.

Table 2.1   Factors influencing WASH behaviour

Factor	Example – promotion of hand washing
Specific knowledge	Knowing when to wash hands, and being aware that people carry "invisible" faeces on their hands
Knowledge of key WASH skills	Knowing how to wash hands properly
Availability of key supplies and services	Access to the needed water, and soap or ash for washing
Perceptions of community norms (i.e. what people think others who are important to them believe they should do)	Being aware of what family or friends would think of someone coming to the table with unwashed hands
Anticipated and actual consequences for doing or not doing the behaviour	Anticipating the possibility of infection if hands are not washed properly

Because it can be difficult to get people to change their WASH practices, this guides suggests two fundamental ways to approach behaviour change; these are to make it possible and negotiate improved practice.

These approaches, discussed below, will help to encourage small improvements that can significantly improve the lives and livelihoods of PLHIV and their families.

2.8.1   Make it possible

Encouraging a householder with limited resources to adopt the ideal practice immediately is often a recipe for failure, because people rarely go directly from their current practice to the ideal practice. For example, a person is unlikely to go from not washing their hands to washing them with soap at the five critical times, or from drinking water from a contaminated source to drinking water from a protected source and storing it in a jerry can with a spigot. A more effective approach for a programme is to identify a few feasible and effective actions that move closer to the ideal, and will have a positive effect on household and public health. Programmes can promote such actions – referred to as "small doable actions" (see Box 2.2 and Annex 4).

Box 2.2   What is a small doable action?

In the context of WASH, a small doable action is a behaviour that, when practiced consistently and correctly, will lead to improvement in household and public health (in this case, reducing diarrhoea). The action is one that is considered feasible by the householder, from that person's point of view, when taking into account the current practice, the available resources and the particular social context. Although the behaviour may not be an "ideal practice", households are likely to adopt this small action because it will be seen as feasible within the local context, whereas the ideal may seem out of reach.

Identifying small doable actions involves imagining a spectrum, with the worst behaviour at one end and the ideal practice at the other. Somewhere on the spectrum is a point (the minimum requirement) at which practice is consistent and will have a positive public health outcome. If current practice falls below that minimum requirement, then small doable actions are needed to move people towards the ideal practice, as illustrated in Box 2.3.

Box 2.3   Illustrative small doable actions for safe water treatment and storage

- Use a 20 l jerry can with a cover to store drinking water.

- Attach the cover to the jerry can with a string to keep it off the floor.

- Wash the jerry can and its cover with soap and water every day.

- Treat drinking water in the jerry can with a chlorine generating product.

- Pour water from the jerry can into a clean cup or glass; alternatively, pour it into a clean jug with a cover and then pour it into a clean glass.

- Do NOT touch the jerry can on the inside or on the rim with hands.

2.8.2   Negotiate improved practice

Those wishing to influence behaviour must work with household members to solve problems and get them to try to improve their WASH practices. This is called "negotiating improved practice". As shown in Table 2.1, householders need not only key information, but also skills, access to required supplies, social acceptance and confidence that they can succeed in practising the new behaviours. The home visitor, counsellor, family member or clinician must assess what the current barriers are to each WASH practice and how they can be overcome. The person then needs to negotiate a commitment to try a few practices that seem feasible, worth changing and safe, from the point of view of the householder (rather than from someone else's assessment of what is important).

To negotiate improved practice, ask questions such as those listed below (substituting other issues, as necessary):

- **What makes it hard to** … wash your hands with running water and soap after defecation, before preparing food, and before eating or feeding others?

- **What would make it easier to** … wash your hands with running water and soap after defecation, before preparing food, and before eating or feeding others?

- **Who approves of you spending time and resources to** … wash your hands with running water and soap after defecation, before preparing food, and before eating or feeding others?

The responses to these questions will help to identify problems, fears and barriers to change, and how change could be brought about. This information can be used in programme design, as it will highlight current knowledge and skills, relevant social factors, cultural practices, and access to products and services.

Other tools to support the process of changing behaviour include:

- practical, simple tools that can be used by community workers with good facilitation skills to engage communities in dialogue; for example, participatory hygiene and sanitation transformation (PHAST) – a participatory approach for promoting improved sanitation;[1]

- participatory tools for hygiene promotion programming, adapted from the PHAST methodology by the International Federation of the Red Cross and Red Crescent Societies;

- behaviour change tools on web sites from organizations such as the Core Group,[2] the United States Agency for International Development/Hygiene Improvement Project (USAID/HIP)[3] and the Manoff Group.[4]

It is not possible to change everything at once. Those wishing to change behaviour should identify two or three improved practices, and negotiate with the householder to try these practices until the next visit.

---

[1] http://www.who.int/water_sanitation_health/hygiene/envsan/phastep/en
[2] http://www.coregroup.org
[3] http://www.hip.watsan.net
[4] http://www.manoffgroup.com

3 Including WASH in national HIV/AIDS policies and related materials

Many countries have written materials to help health professionals to develop HIV programmes. These materials include policies, strategies, guidelines, standards, action plans, handbooks and training manuals. Some countries have also produced specific guidance for different aspects of HIV prevention, care and support, including guidelines for home-based care, orphans and vulnerable children, counselling and testing, food and nutrition, and PMTCT.

The team paid special attention to obtaining available materials from several countries with a high prevalence of HIV/AIDS. The types of materials differed between countries.

The team reviewed 30 HIV policy-related documents from 14 countries (Cambodia, Ethiopia, Guyana, Haiti, India, Kenya, Malawi, Namibia, Rwanda, South Africa, Tanzania, Vietnam, Zambia and Zimbabwe). The WASH areas most frequently addressed were safe drinking water and safe food consumption. A few documents mentioned hand washing, faeces disposal and personal hygiene, but this material was often located in the background information. No document mentioned anything about water quantity or storage, menstrual blood management, or adaptation of sanitation and water supply systems for people with mobility restrictions. Also, these documents provided almost no information on how to practise WASH actions. Countries often have comprehensive information on WASH actions available, but contained in more general health or environmental health documents. In such cases, the country should link these health documents more comprehensively with HIV policy documents.

The two standards reviewed (from Zimbabwe in 2004 and Namibia in 2008[1]) were the most explicit in listing specific WASH behaviours. Zambia's nutrition guidelines also covered many WASH behaviours in some detail. A review of home-based care guidelines for a 2007 WASH–HIV integration meeting in Malawi found that Zimbabwe's policy was the most comprehensive in integrating WASH and HIV, and that the country's guidelines have some useful material and graphics, which can be adapted for use in other countries. Malawi's home-based care guidelines provided greater detail than most on using safe water and keeping the environment clean. Malawi's sanitation policy suggested that programmes be HIV and AIDS

---

[1] http://www.c-changeproject.org/where-we-work/namibia

aware. Kenya has several levels of HIV policy and guidance, and its handbook for home-based care workers on HIV care and support provides useful and specific information, actions and standards for WASH. In documents from other countries, language was very general; for example, documents suggested that providers and HIV-affected families maintain personal hygiene and perhaps drink boiled or "clean" water, but generally failed to give specific guidance.

Clearly, better guidance and recommendations on WASH are needed in national HIV guidelines for home-based care, orphans and vulnerable children, food and nutrition, PMTCT, etc. Generally, there is a need for guidance to be more specific and actionable. The sections below highlight how guidelines can be modified to provide greater emphasis on WASH; they suggest specific language to include, particularly for country policies and guidance.

3.1 Integrating WASH into global HIV/AIDS policy and guidance

Key agencies such as UNAIDS, USAID and WHO have developed key reference documents that are used by national AIDS programmes and NGOs to set local policy and guidance. To help countries integrate WASH into HIV policies, these agencies also need to integrate WASH into their key reference documents. The types of actions that should be taken at this global level are listed below.

- Modify reference documents used to develop country policies and guidelines.

  - Include necessary WASH behaviours in a minimum package of services for HIV prevention and treatment, and in a counselling sheet; also, include WASH supplies (e.g. soap, hypochlorite solution, gloves and plastic sheeting) in kits given to PLHIV. Be specific; for example, list key WASH practices and any equipment or supplies needed, and explain how to do each practice. Include WASH in monitoring and recording forms.

- Revise minimum packages, home-based care kits, school-based HIV education kits, indicator lists and monitoring forms to include WASH.

  - For policies, provide a general description of what a WASH package should contain.

  - For guidelines, provide specific descriptions of WASH topics.

  - For standards, explain each WASH practice in detail so that providers know what to do, and how to instruct householders in WASH practices.

- Ensure that policies and guidelines suggest environmental health collaboration at all levels, as part of the multisectoral focus.
  - The multisectoral focus could include water, sanitation and education programme managers, and others as appropriate.
- Learn from other multisectoral interventions.
  - Other guidelines (e.g. those on food and nutrition security) may be useful, as they may already have highlighted important WASH behaviours.
  - Ensure that WASH elements, indicators and so on are integrated into activities related to food and nutrition security.
  - Promote a WASH minimum package for home-based care and support services. The package should emphasize key hygiene behaviours, and the products and infrastructure needed to put these into practice, such as latrines, hand-washing stations, soap and chlorine solution.
- Develop a list of key WASH behaviours for PLHIV.
  - Develop generic assessment and counselling tools on the WASH behaviours for PLHIV.

3.2 Integrating WASH into country HIV/AIDS policy and guidance

This section aims to help countries identify where and how to include specific language on WASH in guidance documents. The aim is to minimize the spread of diarrhoea throughout HIV-affected communities and beyond.

It is not necessary to develop a free-standing WASH and HIV policy; instead, it is best to integrate WASH policies and guidance into overall HIV policies, whether general HIV or area specific (e.g. orphans and vulnerable children, home-based care and PMTCT).

Provide a framework for integrating evidence-based WASH approaches into HIV/AIDS policies and guidelines. To provide further support to the various groups (e.g. PLHIV, orphans and vulnerable children, and their families), foster links with other programmes that address issues, such as water, and sanitation insecurity and needs in targeted populations, whether or not these programmes are health related. Box 3.1 provides criteria that can be used to assess the extent of WASH considerations in current policy documents.

| Box 3.1 | Criteria for assessing and improving the WASH component of country policies, guidelines and handbooks |

Box 3.1   Criteria for assessing and improving the WASH component of country policies, guidelines and handbooks

The overall objective of the criteria given below is to assess how well (if at all) WASH is included in national policies, guidelines and handbooks. The results of the assessment can be used to add or improve the materials, as appropriate.

Definitions

The following definitions are provided to clarify the general content of policies and guidelines, to guide the assessment or modification of documents.

Policies for HIV/AIDS are generally national or regional documents that state a set of basic principles and associated guidelines that were formulated and are enforced by the governing body. Their purpose is to influence and determine decisions, actions and other matters.

Guidelines aim to streamline particular processes according to a set routine. By definition, guidelines are not mandatory (whereas protocols generally are mandatory). Guidelines are issued or adopted by an organization (governmental or private) to make the actions of its employees more predictable and presumably of higher quality.

Standards are technical specifications or procedures that lay out characteristics of a product or procedure (e.g. levels of quality, performance, safety or dimensions).

Handbooks provide information to supplement guidelines; they specify processes further, and often include job aids or counselling tools to ensure that processes are implemented properly.

Assessment

Follow the steps listed below to assess documents for their inclusion of WASH.

Step 1 – If possible, obtain both printed and electronic versions of any documents. If these are not available, work with the printed documents only.

Step 2 – Start with the table of contents and chapter headings. If the electronic version is available, do a word search (use the "find" function; if necessary, use the "help" function to work out how to use the "find" function). Otherwise, visually scan the table of contents (TOC) and headings for the following key words:

- water, drinking, sanitation, toilet, latrine, hand washing, hygiene, faeces (or feces) and diarrhoea (or diarrhea).

Step 3 – Highlight these words in the TOC and headings.

Step 4 – Using the TOC and headings, locate the sections in the document that contain the key words.

Step 5 – Evaluate the descriptions and statements associated with the key words.

Assess the description or entry by asking whether the information is sufficiently detailed and specific to:

- precisely describe policy or guide a practitioner to implement the policy or practice
- serve as a recipe or formula
- guide choices, when decisions are required or several options are available.

Step 6 – Scan the document again and note where entries should be added.

Improvement

Revise the document as necessary. Appropriate places for change include any mentions of nutrition, feeding, supplementary feeding, home hygiene, personal hygiene, care and support, home-based care, PMTCT, and counselling and testing.

Countries are welcome to add text from this document – particularly from the sections on priority WASH practices for national programmes – to appropriate sections. Further guidance is given in section 3.3.

3.3 Improving WASH guidance

The following sections provide suggestions for how countries can improve WASH guidance when writing or revising HIV-related policies, guidelines and handbooks.

3.2.1 Water access

Care and support guidelines should identify technologies to gather water more easily; for example, lengthening pump handles or installing cement platforms that children can stand on to pump water. Guidelines should also identify water-saving techniques and describe how to install them. For example, care and support guidelines in resource-poor areas should include instructions on collecting rain water and constructing a tippy tap.

3.2.2 Water quantity

National HIV/AIDS guidelines should include estimates of water needed by HIV-affected households; as described in section 1.2, these are greater than the "basic access" estimate of 20 litres per person per day for the general population (WHO, 2006). Table 1.1 (see section 1.2) specifies quantities of water by activity.

Home-based care guidelines should include a section on the amount of water needed to keep PLHIV and their environment clean. This section should include an estimate of the quantity of water needed for the specific area, as well as information on what to clean and how to clean it.

Care and support guidelines should provide specifications for water collection technologies, such as water conservation and rainwater catchment.

3.2.3 Water quality

Guidelines and training materials for care providers should include:

- detailed instructions on water treatment techniques and on proper storage and handling to reduce the potential for recontamination (as described in sections 2.1 and 2.2);

- information on the need for ART to be distributed in conjunction with sodium hypochlorite solution or other water-treatment options to ensure that medicines are taken with clean water;

- information on the need for a preventive care package distributed to PLHIV to include

  – a covered water vessel with a tap (if commonly available; and typical and locally made if possible, to avoid stigmatization);

  – oral rehydration salts, soap or other evidence-based interventions.

Guidelines for the community at large should promote the same container and water-treatment product that is included in ART distribution. Alternatively, such guidelines can promote broader social marketing of water disinfection products.

3.2.4 Sanitation access

National guidelines on sanitation access for PLHIV should meet the requirements listed below.

- Identify and promote sanitary options for defecation.

- Promote construction of improved pit latrines at the household level where there is sufficient space. Where space is limited, as in urban areas, promote a feasible option (based on contextual and environmental factors) such as:

  – condominial latrines[1] connected to a shared septic tank or system

  – privately managed pay-for-use public toilets

  – above-ground latrines.

---

[1] Condominal latrines are those used by residents of a housing block, and typically involve consultations and continuing interactions between users and agencies during planning and implementation.

- Promote client-friendly latrines in the household that incorporate the following suggestions (see sections 2.3 and 2.4):
  - an entrance to the latrine that is wide enough to accommodate more than one person, so that another person can assist an unstable user;
  - assistive devices;
  - natural light and adequate ventilation;
  - bedside commodes, bedpans or squat pots;
  - a hand-washing facility with soap or soap substitute (ash) near the latrine.

Also provide detailed instructions on keeping the person, house and surrounding environment clean.

3.2.5 Sanitation, hygiene and hand-washing knowledge and practice

All care and support guidelines and training should include a comprehensive water, sanitation and hygiene component that comprises:

- guidance and technologies on hand washing in water-scarce settings;
- critical times for hand washing and proper technique;
- soap substitutes;
- proper disposal of waste water;
- proper use and maintenance of water and sanitation facilities;
- household water treatment and safe storage;
- clear communication of risks associated with, and protective measures required for, handling of faeces (e.g. when bathing clients and laundering soiled bedding or clothing).

Promotion materials for care and support programmes should include visual materials that are suitable for low-literacy audiences. These should be distributed to caregivers and others who interact with HIV-affected households.

All nutrition guidelines for care and support programmes should include information on WASH because diarrhoea prevents PLHIV from absorbing ART and essential nutrients.

4 Language to use when including WASH in national HIV/AIDS policies and related materials

Chapter 3 provided suggestions for topic areas to include when revising HIV policies, guidelines and handbooks. This chapter provides examples of specific language that can be used to modify HIV/AIDS policies and related materials, using safe drinking water as an example.

4.1 Types of material

4.1.1 Policies

In a national policy, existing text might read:

- *All HIV-infected persons should drink safe water or all households without safe water should boil water for PLHIV to consume.*

An improvement to this text would be to add:

- *All HIV-affected households should treat all drinking water and store the treated water in a narrow mouthed, covered container.*

4.1.2 Guidelines

The text in national guidelines would include the text above from the policy, but include more details about safe hygiene practices. Thus, the revised text in national guidelines might read:

- *Any containers provided at no cost should be those that are commonly used and readily available in the marketplace. A container with a spigot is ideal but is not always feasible for households. Avoid items that are available only to PLHIV, because they identify recipients as HIV-positive and may be stigmatizing.*

- *Sodium hypochlorite solution or tablets are the ideal water treatment methods, because the residual chlorine will protect the water from recontamination for 24 hours, but any of the four effective methods – hypochlorite solution or chlorination, solar disinfection, filtration and boiling – are acceptable.*

4.1.3   Standards of practice

National standards of practice should delineate the essentials of delivering WASH in HIV/AIDS settings at various practice levels and settings. For example, they may include performance expectations for individuals responsible for WASH or HIV programming (e.g. nurses, volunteers and teachers), professional standards and so on. National standards should repeat the guidelines but should also include detailed instructions for treating water by each method. This language can be adapted from section 2.1.

4.1.4   Handbooks

Handbooks should repeat the language from the standards, but should also include counselling tools and job aids for treating and safely storing drinking water.

4.2   Sample text

This section provides text that could be included in its entirety, or adapted and inserted into different documents such as guidelines, standards and handbooks.

Integrating WASH into HIV care and support settings

Many life-threatening opportunistic infections are caused by exposure to unsafe water, inadequate sanitation and poor hygiene. Diarrhoea, a very common symptom that can occur throughout the course of HIV/AIDS, affects 90% of PLHIV and results in significant morbidity and mortality, especially in HIV-infected children.

At least 30% of diarrhoeal diseases could be prevented through integrated programmes that involve providing water treatment and safe storage, safe disposal of faeces, and promotion of key hygiene practices. HIV/AIDS programmes should consider building links among the health, water and sanitation sectors to improve the number of safe water supply points and latrines that are accessible and close to where they are needed.

Safe drinking water

HIV/AIDS programmes are encouraged to ensure that PLHIV in facility-based care settings have access to sufficient safe drinking water and in communities that lack a reliable source of safe water, PLHIV are supported with household water treatment and safe storage methods. Several technologies are available for treating water in the home – they include chlorination, use of various types of filters, proper boiling, SODIS using heat and UV radiation, and combined chemical coagulation, flocculation and disinfection.

Hand washing

Washing hands at critical times, with soap and proper technique, is the most important hygiene measure to be integrated across all HIV/AIDS programmes. Although hand-washing studies are limited in PLHIV, data support the benefits of hand washing in the general population; for example, the practice reduced diarrhoea in Bangladeshi adults by 62% (Shahid et al., 1996) and by 53% in children in Pakistan (Luby et al., 2004).

Programmes should at least provide guidance and training on washing hands and proper technique. Also, they should place hand-washing stations with soap (or soap substitute, such as ash) in facilities, community care points and in the household. Some programmes in water-scarce situations should consider using a tippy tap; that is, a simple plastic jug, gourd or vessel made from local material that regulates the flow of water, to allow for hand washing with a very small quantity of water.

Sanitation

In many countries, people lack access to basic sanitation systems; therefore, it is important to focus on simple efforts (e.g. safe handling and disposal of faeces) that have the biggest health implications. Disposing of faeces safely, keeping faeces away from flies and other insects, and preventing faecal contamination of water supplies can greatly reduce the spread of diseases. However, where people lack easy access to latrines, they will often resort to open defecation methods.

Although HIV programmes have not traditionally funded the construction of simple, on-site waste disposal systems such as latrines, many sanitation interventions that will benefit PLHIV and their families can be supported. For example, health workers, caregivers, family members and PLHIV need to learn how to build a latrine and how to use existing latrines safely. Further, installing poles or stools in a latrine will help weak PLHIV to use the latrine. If a latrine is not available, faeces must be collected in a bedpan and buried away from the facility, clinic or home, and away from where animals can dig it up. Similarly, if a client is weak, less mobile or bedbound, and cannot use a latrine, programmes can ensure access to simple commodes or bedpans that can be used by PLHIV to defecate in the bed or house; the faeces can then be disposed of, as described above, by caregivers.

Adult care programmes need to ensure that PLHIV with diarrhoea are supported to protect their skin, sheets, clothing and mattress from becoming soiled with faeces. Strategies such as placing a plastic sheet covered by paper or a cloth under the client's buttocks are very simple and cost-effective measures that can ease the caregiving burden.

Personal, nutritional and environmental hygiene

Ensuring personal, nutritional and environmental hygiene is essential to reducing the infectious disease burden experienced by PLHIV. Diseases related to water and sanitation can be effectively reduced by a combination of:

- improved water treatment and handling
- faeces removal
- personal hygiene (i.e. PLHIV and health worker hygiene and cleanliness)
- food hygiene (i.e. safe cooking, mixing, storage and disposal of food)
- ensuring a hygienic environment in clinics and in homes.

In particular, caregivers and volunteers involved in home-based care require hygiene education; thus, this type of information must be included in home-based care training.

5 Programme approaches for WASH–HIV integration

Comprehensive water, sanitation and hygiene strategies include a wide range of interventions to improve the quality of life for PLHIV and their families. These interventions are not specific to any one setting or location, and are generally delivered through the home, community, school or facility. WASH interventions cannot be standardized for all situations and countries, because specific methods of implementing WASH will vary. Therefore, this chapter presents a "menu" of interventions that could be considered. The WASH components to be implemented should be selected and prioritized locally; the components selected should be consistent with national guidelines.

National programme managers are encouraged to:

- understand the essential WASH actions for diarrhoeal disease prevention and use this information to determine what types of WASH approaches already exist in country programmes (HIV or otherwise);

- examine the types of potential WASH approaches, the cost of these approaches and which programmes might fit best into HIV/AIDS programming in each country;

- to prioritize these activities for integration into country plans.

Table 5.1 lists the different programme approaches and, in each case, provides examples and links to relevant web sites.

Table 5.1   Illustrative programme approaches

Programme approaches	Examples/links
Integrate or mainstream WASH as an issue spanning all intervention areas (OVC, PMTCT, CT, etc.)	Integrate WASH into existing community-based approaches, such as HBC and community-based care, post-test clubs, PMTCT/HBC support groups, behaviour-change communication strategies and campaigns, etc. Programmes can more easily be included in mainstream HBC and community-based care by distributing a WASH household assessment tool for use by all who do home visits. The tool can be used to quickly identify existing WASH conditions and recommendations for practical "small doable actions". Based on assessment, and resources and support in the community, integrate WASH into all HIV/AIDS service-delivery training for providers, caregivers, community health workers, etc. Make available appropriate curriculum for adaptation and integration, and job aids: • 'Train-the-trainer' guide and participant manual for integrating wash into home-based care. http://www.hip.watsan.net/page/2708 • Pictorial tool and counselling cards for HBC givers in Ethiopia, used to counsel community and family members on WASH actions. http://www.hip.watsan.net/page/2708
Build NGO and government capacity	Build the capacity of WASH and HIV/AIDS programmes to deliver in-country technical assistance, supervision, planning and training. USAID is currently implementing this approach in Ethiopia and Uganda across sectors to improve WASH and HIV/AIDS programmes. See case studies in section 5.3.
Integrate WASH training into all HIV/AIDS service delivery trainings	CDC has developed training resources that can be easily adapted locally. Topics covered are: • safe water treatment and storage (at least 4 hours of training) • hand washing at critical times, and with proper technique and other personal hygiene measures (at least 4 hours of training) http://www.cdc.gov/safewater/publications_pages/fact_sheets/SWSTrainingGuidNurses.pdf http://www.cdc.gov/safewater/publications_pages/fact_sheets/SWSCurriculumNurses.pdf http://www.shea-online.org/Assets/files/IHI_Hand_Hygiene.pdf Training is also essential in other aspects of WASH: • promoting improved sanitation (at least 4 hours of training) • food hygiene (at least 2 hours of training) • personal and environmental cleanliness (at least 2 hours of training).
Develop and use curricula, behaviour change, and counselling tools and materials	Develop supplements or integrate WASH themes into: • participant manuals; • trainer manuals; • flipcharts; • information education and communication materials, especially reminder materials for PLHIV homes; and • pocket cards for health workers to use to help them remember key points. Examples of available professional training and school-based curricula are found in the case studies in section 5.3.

Table 5.1 *continued*

Programme approaches	Examples/links
Implement a basic care package through the clinic system	In the package of commodities given to HIV-positive and PMTCT clients, include a hypochlorite product, a container (of a type available locally) and soap, with accompanying hygiene education, reinforcement and follow-up. The package represents evidence-based practices that can help to maintain PLHIV health. Other commodities may include condoms, ORT, multivitamins and cotrimoxazole. Health-care providers are trained in how to educate and counsel clients on the kit.
Include a comprehensive WASH package for adult PLHIV and families in the home setting	In the package of commodities given to adult PHLIV and families in the home setting, include a hypochlorite product, a container (of a type available locally) and soap, with accompanying hygiene education; instructions on making devices for hand washing with limited water and bedpans for facilitating safe disposal of faeces; tips for making latrine use easier for PLHIV (especially those with limited mobility); gloves; and plastic sheeting.
Ensure adequate supply of essential hygiene commodities	Safe water treatment and storage commodities include: • treatment products (hypochlorite solution or tablets, filters, etc. for water purification); • 1–2 l transparent plastic bottles appropriate for SODIS; • safe water storage containers (clay pot, jerry can or container with a spigot), lids and dippers; and • spigot or tap available in the local market. http://www.cdc.gov/safewater/publications_pages/proven.pdf http://www.cdc.gov/safewater/publications_pages/options-sodis.pdf http://www.cdc.gov/safewater/publications_pages/fact_sheets/SWSCurriculumNurses.pdf Hand-washing commodities include: • soap and alternative local products, such as ash; • materials for making a tippy tap, such as a plastic jug, gourd or local material with spigot or opening (to provide a slow stream of water); and rope; http://www.cdc.gov/safewater/publications_pages/tippy-tap.pdf • hand-washing stations in health facilities or schools (Parker et al., 2006; O'Reilly et al., 2008). Commodities for safe handling and disposal of faeces, urine and menstrual blood include: • rubber, mackintosh or plastic sheets to protect linen, mattresses and skin; • a bedpan or bedside structure (i.e. a commode) to help clients who are unable to get to a latrine or toilet (these items should be created with local materials – for both infants and adults) • clean cloth, diapers and plastic pants for incontinent clients (infants and adults) • gloves for safely handling faeces and body fluids • hygiene stations (for hand washing with soap or ash) – if necessary, can create a tippy tap

Table 5.1 *continued*

Programme approaches	Examples/links
	• sanitation platforms for latrines.
	Food hygiene commodities include:
	• treated water for preparation of nutrition products (e.g. complementary foods, formula);
	• sanitizing food or formula preparation vessels, and washing and treating raw fruits and vegetables; and
	• hygiene stations (for hand washing with soap) – if necessary, can create a tippy tap.
	Personal cleanliness and environmental hygiene commodities include:
	• clean cloth for daily bathing, hygiene, etc.;
	• bags for collecting and disposing of waste; and
	• hygiene stations (for hand washing with soap) – if necessary, can create a tippy tap.
Appropriate behaviour change, communication and counselling	Commodities are only effective if they are used correctly and consistently; therefore, accompany all commodity distribution with adequate education, follow-up, reinforcement and monitoring. This may include clinic-based education, home visits, peer support groups, etc.
Support supervision	Follow up with providers or teachers, staff, etc. to reinforce improved WASH behaviours. Add to or develop and use job aids, supervision checklists and tools to improve the performance monitoring of providers, teachers, etc. Checklists should include a check of presence of hand-washing station with signs of use, latrine with signs of use and presence of soap. Distribute "how to" sheets (e.g. on making a tippy tap) as part of monitoring.
Recruit and fund coordinator	Support a local WASH-integration coordinator who is dedicated to working with partners to integrate hygiene into the HIV/AIDS programme.
Explore options for increasing access to water and sanitation infrastructure	Within the local country context, identify partners already working in water and sanitation, and explore possibilities for leveraging water and sanitation infrastructure. Start by examining UNICEF and World Bank operations to see if existing programmes to support water and sanitation infrastructure will also support WASH for HIV goals.
Support national committees on WASH and HIV/AIDS	Form national steering committees to improve programming and leadership on WASH and HIV/AIDS. For example, the Government of Uganda has formed a National Working Group on Hygiene Improvement and HIV/AIDS to guide the technical mainstreaming of WASH and HIV with donor support.

AIDS, acquired immunodeficiency virus; CDC, Centers for Disease Control and Prevention; CT, counselling and testing; HBC, home-based care; HIV, human immunodeficiency virus; ORT, oral rehydration therapy; OVC, orphans and vulnerable children; NGO, nongovernmental organization; PLHIV, people living with HIV; PMTCT, prevention of mother-to-child transmission; SODIS, solar disinfection; USAID, United States Agency for International Development; WASH, water, sanitation and hygiene.

5.1   Coordination with water and sanitation sectors

HIV and AIDS are often characterized as health issues and are therefore not integrated into plans and activities of other sectors. In particular, ministries of health, and ministries of water or sanitation rarely coordinate or develop joint plans. Even within NGOs, managers of water, sanitation and health programmes are often unaware of one other's strategic planning – even health and HIV programme managers are often strangers to one another.

Yet, to remain healthy, everyone (and especially those living with HIV) needs access to water and sanitation services, and needs to practice good hygiene. Further, these services must be accessible, affordable and reliable. Households that have lost their primary income generators are less able to pay water or latrine fees; also, fewer able-bodied people in households mean fewer people available to manage water and sanitation activities in the community (Franks & Cleaver, 2002).

5.1.1   Integrating HIV considerations into water supply and sanitation activities

As noted throughout this document, people affected by HIV and AIDS have greater need of water and sanitation services than the general population. The burden of HIV care and support falls largely on the most vulnerable: sick people, female caregivers (who are often elderly) and children (who are often most affected by insufficient water supply and sanitation). Further, as documented by a case study in Tanzania, labour-poor households, youth-headed households and elderly women are all under-represented on the water and sanitation committees where decisions are made (Kamminga & Wegelin-Schuringa, 2005).

Most WASH-related programmes do not address HIV/AIDS (Kamminga & Wegelin-Schuringa, 2005), either from the human resource perspective (even though high HIV prevalence can decimate staffing within the water and sanitation sectors) or from the hardware standpoint (i.e. they fail to apply the technological innovations that could improve access to services). Thus, integrating HIV into the water and sanitation sectors must deal with the following two parallel spheres simultaneously:

- protecting sectoral human resources through HIV prevention and mitigation programmes (not addressed by this document);

- considering the special hardware needs of those affected by HIV in WASH programmes and activities; examples of the latter might include

    - lengthening pump handles to make it easier to pump water

    - building wells or latrines closer to HIV-affected households

    - building ramps or platforms for easier access.

Water and sanitation technologies are generally designed for able-bodied people who can operate, maintain and walk to the facilities (UN-HABITAT, 2007). The HIV/AIDS context demands new paradigms, such as placing facilities near people who are too weak to walk long distances, and designing water points and latrines in ways that consider the special needs of PLHIV and their families.

Finally, if PLHIV are unable to participate in planning, decision-making and implementation, this will limit consideration of PLHIV-specific water and sanitation needs. In the HIV context, communities must have the ability to finance and manage water supply and sanitation changes; also, water and sanitation sectors must strive to ensure that installations are robust, affordable and can be sustained without reliance on a declining pool of skilled outsiders (Kamminga & Wegelin-Schuringa, 2005).

Table 5.2 describes some activities the water and sanitation sectors can include when planning infrastructure and education programmes with communities.

Table 5.2   Suggestions for integrating HIV considerations into water and sanitation sector plans and programmes

Planning
Consider HIV needs when developing water and sanitation policies, planning, regulation, service delivery and provision.
Develop strategic partnerships with other sectors or stakeholders (e.g. HIV/AIDS, HBC providers) to address the most vulnerable: women, children and the elderly.
Develop guidelines and strategies to integrate HIV/AIDS awareness into all water and sanitation sectoral projects. Create an institutional framework that is HIV-sensitive, to ensure that poorer communities that experience difficulty in paying for services have access to improved water sources.
Identify and address issues specific to HIV-infected and affected families, such as needs for additional quantity of water, latrine access, etc.
Map access to water and sanitation points, and target areas of HIV prevalence or vulnerability when constructing new water and sanitation points.
Integrate PLHIV and affected family perspectives into community water management and planning schemes, by including PLHIV and community care organization representatives in decision making.

Technology
Develop and promote new water-collection technologies and strategies to bring water closer to the home (e.g. rainwater catchment systems, ergonomic pump designs using local materials).
Recommend hand-washing stations as part of a twin design for all latrine construction.
Promote water-saving technologies such as tippy taps for washing hands.
Include minimum standards for latrines that allow for an assistant to accompany the PLHIV to the latrine, and options for outfitting latrines with support poles, squatting stools or seats for greater comfort.

Community access
Assess effects of inability to pay on water and sanitation systems; develop alternative structures, such as focused subsidies, to ensure that vulnerable households have access to water and toilets/latrines.
Promote community participation to provide support to vulnerable groups digging the pit, constructing the superstructure.

Education
Incorporate information on the special needs of PLHIV and other vulnerable populations into education and training for water and sanitation sectors.
Assess how to support communities to access safe water supply sanitation and hygiene education to mitigate the impact of HIV/AIDS and to support community care to those infected and affected.

AIDS, acquired immunodeficiency virus; HBC, home-based care; HIV, human immunodeficiency virus; PLHIV, people living with HIV; WASH, water, sanitation and hygiene.

5.2   Monitoring and evaluation

To reduce diarrhoeal disease and make other improvements for families affected by HIV, donors and programme managers must clearly articulate programme objectives and relevant ways of measuring those objectives.

This section contains a set of illustrative indicators and objectives that can be used to measure integration activities.

Programmes can select or adapt the illustrative indicators listed below depending on the scope of integration activities and the extent to which the programme can monitor them. The indicators, organized by objective, are as follows:

- *Objective 1* – Increased policy support for integrating WASH into HIV programmes.

- *Objective 2* – Increased institutional capacity to plan, implement and evaluate the integration of WASH into HIV programmes in communities and households.

- *Objective 3* – Increased adoption of WASH practices in households of PLHIV and households affected by HIV.

Table 5.3 shows the indicators for each of these objectives.

Table 5.3   Illustrative indicators and objectives that can be used to measure integration activities

Illustrative indicators

Objective 1 – Increased policy support for integrating WASH into HIV programmes

Appropriate specifications of WASH elements that should be included in HIV guidance and policy are:
- hand washing, food safety, safe water handling and treatment, and management of sanitation and faeces in OVC;
- PMTCT;
- nutrition and food security;
- ART;
- HBC and community-based care,
- general HIV-related documents – policies, standards, guidelines and handbooks; and
- percentage of HIV budget dedicated to WASH-related activities or commodities (which may or may not be chosen for inclusion).

Objective 2 – Increased institutional capacity to plan, implement and evaluate the integration of WASH into HIV programmes in communities and households

Appropriate specifications for increasing the institutional capacity to plan, implement and evaluate the integration of WASH into HIV programmes are:
- percentage of targeted organizations, ministries or bureaux reporting modifications that include WASH in their current HIV programming;
- number of HIV providers by cadre (HBC workers, community health workers, PMTCT counsellors, OVC providers, nutrition counsellors, VCT counsellors, etc.) trained in
  - WASH essentials
  - negotiating behaviour change;
- percentage of trained HIV providers who have mastered WASH knowledge and skills;
- percentage of trained HIV providers who perform WASH competencies according to established standards;
- percentage of targeted organizations who have modified follow-up supervision and monitoring to include WASH elements;
- percentage of targeted organizations, ministries and bureaux reporting collaboration of HIV programmes with WASH programmes;
- percentage of targeted organizations, ministries and bureaux with joint documents, joint decisions and policies, work plans, etc.;
- percentage of targeted organizations mapping or assessing communities to determine which organizations are providing WASH improvement as part of their planning assessments;
- percentage of antistigma sessions that address some element of water and sanitation stigma (e.g. HIV-infected people being unable to use common water sources or shared latrines);
- percentage of households enrolled in HBC receiving minimum package of services that include key WASH elements of care and counselling (reported by householder or by provider (forms); and
- percentage of households enrolled in HBC receiving HBC kit that includes WASH-related supplies, reported by householder or by provider (forms).

Objective 3 – Increased adoption of WASH practices in households of PLHIV and households affected by HIV

Appropriate specifications for increasing the adoption of WASH practices in households of PLHIV and households affected by HIV are summarized below.

Hand washing

Data first collected at household level, then calculated as percentage of households.

Table 5.3 *continued*

- Percentage of targeted households with a designated place for hand washing (hand-washing station) commonly used by caregiver and client equipped with hand-washing supplies (i.e. water and a local cleansing agent such as soap or ash).
- Is the hand-washing device fixed in one location or movable?
- Person can name at least 2 of 4 critical times to wash hands to prevent diseases.

Safe handling and disposal of faeces

Data first collected at household level, then calculated as percentage of households.

- Presence of latrine in compound or shared between two compounds
    - none;
    - unimproved (no slab, no pit; bucket only); or
    - improved (washable platform, superstructure, cover over pit, 5 m away from house).
- Percentage of latrines in targeted households that are modified to address HIV and mobility issues (stools, grip pole or rope, double chamber for larger latrine, etc.).
- Percentage of targeted households
    - that put children's faeces into a latrine;
    - with a commode or bedpan; and
    - with gloves or bags used to protect caregivers from HIV exposure.

Menstrual management

- Percentage of female clients reporting hygienic disposal of soiled feminine hygiene products.
- Percentage of caregivers reporting appropriate washing of soiled rags used for client menstrual hygiene.

Treatment and safe storage of drinking water at home

Data first collected at household level, then calculated as percentage of households.

- Having a safe water storage container (narrow neck vessel with tightly fitting cover; spigot ideal).
- Reporting sufficient quantity of water available for
    - the PLHIV (and household) to drink
    - the PLHIV to take medications
    - bathing the PLHIV
    - cleaning clothing and bedsheets.

Personal hygiene and household cleanliness

- Percentage of clients that bathed the day before the survey.
- Percentage of targeted households that
    - washed bed linen in the 7 days before survey
    - disposed of solid household waste in protected pit
    - kept domestic animals outside home of the day of survey.

Food hygiene

- Percentage of PLHIV households where
    - available raw meat, poultry or seafood on day of visit is kept separate from raw foods;
    - no cooked food is left standing uncovered more than two hours after being cooked; and fruits and vegetables eaten raw on the day of the interview were washed (with safe water) or fully peeled before consumption.

ART, antiretroviral therapy; HBC, home-based care; HIV, human immunodeficiency virus; OVC, orphans and vulnerable children; PLHIV, people living with HIV; PMTCT, prevention of mother-to-child transmission; VCT, voluntary counselling and testing; WASH, water, sanitation and hygiene.

5.3 Case studies

This section contains practical case studies – snapshots of types of intervention activities that different programmes are trying around the world, to integrate WASH and HIV. USAID/HIP tried to identify a more geographically representative sample of case studies, but most of the examples were located in Africa where HIV/AIDS is most prevalent and where programmes are more advanced.

5.3.1 Ethiopia – integrating WASH into HIV programmes

USAID/HIP created a community of practice (COP) in 2007, comprising six organizations based in Addis Ababa, Ethiopia, all of whom were interested in integrating WASH and HIV. The COP is designed to share experiences and work together to develop programming guidance and tools that can be used to integrate WASH and HIV.

In 2008, the COP compiled a set of small doable actions for key WASH practices and identified areas in which further research in the HIV context was needed. USAID/HIP then conducted research[1] with two COP partners: Catholic Relief Services (CRS) and Save the Children, in Addis Ababa and Oromiya. The results helped to define the gaps – in sanitation practices, treatment and safe storage of drinking water practices, and in a new area, menstrual management practices – and complete the set of small doable actions for the HIV programme context.

In 2009, HIP held a WASH–HIV integration workshop for COP members and other organizations interested in joining the COP. Members of seven organizations attended, with the aim of identifying ways to either integrate WASH considerations into their HIV programmes or integrate HIV considerations into their WASH programmes, using existing assets to achieve the integration. Facilitators and participants discussed tools that have been developed (e.g. job aids and training materials) that are useful and relevant. USAID/HIP will train trainers to cascade WASH activities into these organizations and their programmes, provide job aids for all COP outreach workers, and help to develop indicators for inclusion in monitoring and assessment tools.

In Bahir Dar, USAID/HIP trained a cadre of trainers and then approximately 350 home-based care workers from three organizations who have begun to integrate WASH into their home-based care programmes. The home-based

---

[1] The research involved "trials of improved practices" (TIPs) – a participatory research method that engages selected households to try 1–3 possible recommended behaviours over a 4–8 week period. Researchers visit several times during the period and together with the householders they solve problems, modify behaviours and agree on a set of behaviours that are considered possible by the target audience (given the context and existing resources) and effective in reducing morbidity.

care providers said that, before the USAID/HIP training, they would talk generally about personal hygiene, but did not focus on specific hygiene practices. They appreciated the practical training and could now see how important WASH is for PLHIV, and for orphans and vulnerable children. Since the training, many people have constructed a tippy tap and some have made bedpans from ceramic pots. In addition, the home-based care workers are giving practical instructions on how to wash hands, when to wash hands and the importance of using a latrine.

For more information, contact Julia Rosenbaum, jrosenba@aed.org or Renuka Bery, rbery@aed.org.

5.3.2 Kenya – household water treatment for home-based care workers

The Kenya Red Cross Society is implementing family health home-based care projects targeting PLHIV and other chronically ill people in seven branches countrywide. Key components of the initiative include training communities and community health volunteers in nursing care, and in psychosocial, nutritional and other social support. Through partnerships with various institutions, the programme has managed to increase access to voluntary counselling and testing, ART, treatment services for opportunistic infections, and support for orphans and vulnerable children.

A pilot programme targeted safe household water interventions in 1500 households in Siaya and Kisumu. Households were introduced to water treatment methods and products (filters, PUR, Aquatabs and Watermaker), and trained on the safe water chain, which includes proper transportation, handling, storage, use and reuse of water. Information, education and communication materials were used for hygiene promotion and education, and the programme regularly followed up and monitored the practices.

Because all community members in the project target group were included, the community widely accepted the safe water activities. The programme considered everyone's needs and avoided targeting PLHIV households directly. Most clients were given the chance to try different treatment methods – chlorination was found to be most popular method, followed by filtration and then boiling. The target group reported safe water storage practices; most clients treated drinking water the day before the interview and used appropriate water containers, such as an ordinary clay pot, a plastic jerry can or a modern clay pot. Clients reported adhering to hygiene practices, such as hand washing using correct technique and they correctly identified critical times to wash hands.

For more information, contact Libertad Gonzalez, libertad.gonzalez@ifrc.org or Robert Fraser, robert.fraser@ifrc.org.

5.3.3 Kenya – safe water systems and hand-washing stations in schools

Programme experiences in Kenya demonstrate that unsafe WASH conditions have a detrimental effect on the health of children under five years of age, and on the health, attendance and learning capacities of school-age children, including orphans and vulnerable children. A programme in western Kenya, supported by the United States Government, placed safe water systems and hand-washing stations near primary school kitchens and latrines. Primary school teachers and students were taught correct techniques for hand washing, and water treatment and storage, and students were encouraged to teach their parents improved WASH behaviours. Several organizations – CARE/Kenya, Population Services International (PSI)/Kenya and the CDC – facilitated technical assistance, training and commodity distribution; activities covered included water treatment with bleach, safe storage of treated water and behaviour change communication. An evaluation of this programme documented a 35% decrease in student absentee rates (O'Reilly et al., 2008).

Other examples of school programmes include developing WASH-friendly school guidelines, teacher and student training, integrating WASH into youth clubs and other strategies. UNICEF guidelines promote child-friendly water and sanitation facilities, and hygiene education programmes in all schools.

For more information, see
http://www.cdc.gov/safewater/publications_pages/fact_sheets/Kenya.pdf.

The President's Emergency Plan for AIDS Relief (PEPFAR) web site has resources that can be used in schools and with groups caring for orphans and vulnerable children (see http://www.pepfar.gov).

5.3.4 Malawi – paving the road to health with small doable actions

In 2006, the CRS assessed the WASH component of home-based care supported by WHO in both Zambia and Malawi. The Malawi assessment (Lockwood et al., 2006) found:

- a high prevalence of diarrhoea among home-based care household members;

- a lack of close, available water-supply sources;

- low access to hand-washing facilities and unclean sanitation facilities;

- low levels of treatment of drinking water arising from a false belief that water from the source was safe;

- low levels of WASH education, and a discrepancy between knowledge and behaviour;

- home-based care volunteers not trained or equipped to provide education on water and sanitation.

CRS Malawi worked with WHO and USAID in 2007 to organize a national conference on integrating WASH into home-based care strategies and to mobilize other agencies to think about integration. The October 2007 conference, with more than 50 participants, developed recommendations for integrating WASH activities into home-based care programmes and for integrating HIV considerations into WASH programmes. Malawi partners developed action plans for integrating WASH and HIV.

As part of the conference follow-up, CRS and Dedza Catholic Health Commission developed a pilot project to improve the WASH conditions of home-based care households and community-based childcare centres. The project focused on hand washing, treatment and safe storage of drinking water, and safe disposal of faeces, especially through consistent latrine use. Pilot project activities included:

- training home-based care volunteers and community-based childcare centre caregivers in small, doable WASH actions, and in participatory hygiene and sanitation training (PHAST);
- distributing water treatment products;
- constructing sanitation platform demonstration slabs and tippy taps using locally available materials;
- conducting community education through drama, music and meetings.

Significant changes in knowledge, attitudes and behaviours among targeted home-based care households were recorded one year after the pilot project started. Some of the results are listed below (Senefeld & Powell, 2009).

- Significantly fewer respondents reported that someone in their household had suffered from diarrhoea in the two weeks before the survey (15%) compared to baseline (26%).
- The number of household members who had experienced bloody diarrhoea decreased (from 6% to one case).
- Home-based care household knowledge about washing hands before eating increased (from 81% to 93%), as did washing hands after defecating (from 68% to 87%). Respondents reporting hand-washing facilities almost tripled (from 21% to 60%).
- Home-based care households with treated drinking water almost doubled (from 43% to 84%) and households using a two-cup system to get drinking water increased (from 23% to 56%). A "two-cup system" refers to water being poured into a pitcher or cup, and then poured into a different cup for drinking.

- Half the respondents reported latrines with slabs and the remaining reported an open pit latrine. The number of clean latrine slabs (no visible faecal matter) increased by 14%.

- Health-seeking behaviour increased significantly, with 43% of those with diarrhoea reporting having visited a health centre in response to the diarrhoea (up from 20%).

Performance on almost all project indicators improved during the one-year pilot project. Outcome indicators demonstrated an increase in WASH knowledge, attitudes and practices. These increases contributed to improved health among home-based care household members. This project found that small doable actions for home-based care households are an effective method to improve WASH practices.

For more information, contact Antonia Powell, apowell@mw.saro.crs.org.

5.3.5 Malawi – AIDS drinking water project

In Malawi, 12% of the adult population is infected with HIV, and more than half (59%) of those infected are women. Safe Water International is currently implementing a project in central Malawi that makes drinking water more accessible to HIV-infected people and their families. The project has built rainwater collection tanks (7000 gallon capacity) at three HIV/AIDS treatment centres and is beginning to distribute locally produced sand filters to HIV-affected households.

The project found that the rainwater tanks had a dual purpose: they provided non-contaminated water to clinic clients, but they also motivated clients to come to the clinic. The number of people that attended the health centres once or twice a week increased after the tanks were constructed. In addition, Peace Corps volunteers are developing materials to train villagers to use the sand filter and to teach information about basic WASH practices, such as hand washing with soap, safe water storage, and latrine construction and use.

In June 2009, Safe Water International and home-based care volunteers established some village health centres. They are now working to create a model for a village health care and education programme that incorporates WASH practices and reaches members of the village.

For more information, contact Larry Siegel, lesiegel@cox.net.

5.3.6 South Africa – leveraging external resources for water and sanitation infrastructure

In South Africa, a global development alliance was created to address community water needs in Africa. With support from the Global Environment and Technology Foundation, the Water and Development Alliance contributes to improving water-use efficiency by implementing targeted interventions, increasing access to water supply and sanitation services, and increasing the productive uses of water.

In South Africa, implementing agents are targeting young people and those who are infected with or affected by HIV. The approach involves expanded water reticulation (piped water) in especially deep rural areas in conjunction with hygiene and sanitation behaviour-change programming and training. Funding from PEPFAR is being leveraged to reach up to 25 000 residents in 10 rural villages in Amathole District of the Eastern Cape. In this area, HIV antenatal prevalence is 21%, and 30% of the province has no access to piped water.

For more information, contact Malik Jaffer, mjaffer@usaid.gov.

5.3.7 Uganda – WASH commodities, training and technical assistance

PSI/Uganda is improving water treatment and safe storage, and promoting hand washing with soap by delivering a basic preventive care package for PLHIV and their families. This package of commodities is given through health facilities in coordination with Uganda's Ministry of Health to people who are HIV infected, and participants in ART and PMTCT programmes. The activity includes education on the behaviours and follow-up.

The programme helps to reduce morbidity and mortality caused by opportunistic infections in PLHIV, and to reduce HIV transmission to unborn children and sexual partners. Currently, the basic preventive care package includes identifying PLHIV through family-based counselling and testing, and prolonging and improving the quality of their lives by preventing opportunistic infections. The package combines key informational messages, training and provision of affordable health commodities, including free distribution of a starter kit with:

- two bednets treated with long-lasting insecticide;
- household water treatment chlorine solution, a filter cloth and water vessel;
- condoms;
- health information on how to prevent HIV transmission.

A multichannel communication campaign supports programme implementation by educating PLHIV on how to:

- prevent opportunistic infections;
- live longer and healthier lives through cotrimoxazole prophylaxis;
- prevent diarrhoeal diseases using household water treatment and safe storage;
- prevent malaria by using insecticide treated nets.

The expanded campaign will include palliative care, tuberculosis, HIV and nutrition communication. It will produce education materials (posters, brochures, positive-living client guides and stickers) for PLHIV, health-care providers and counsellors in eight local languages. In partnership with Uganda's Ministry of Health and the Straight Talk Foundation, PSI is producing radio spots and "parent talk" programmes. PSI has trained service providers and peer educators, who are now implementing community activities that reinforce these messages.

PSI now works with 30 HIV care-and-support organizational partners, who have 102 sites implementing the basic preventive care package across Uganda, reaching 250 000 people. Of these sites, 45 have adult clients and distribute condoms, and 8 faith-based organizations work with young infected children. Of the 163 735 kits that have been distributed, nearly 11 000 have been given to children.

For more information, contact Cecilia Kwak, ckwak@psi.org.

5.3.8 Uganda – integrating WASH into HIV/AIDS home-based care programming

Poor WASH practices exert a heavy toll on people living with HIV/AIDS, especially in terms of vulnerability to opportunistic infections and loss of dignity. The additional bouts of diarrhoea and the opportunistic infections experienced by HIV-infected individuals also increase the workload for their caregivers. USAID/HIP is implementing activities to address poor WASH practices in the homes of HIV-infected individuals.

USAID/HIP first conducted focus group discussions and in-depth interviews in urban districts (in Kampala) and rural districts (in Kamuli) to assess hygiene conditions, practices and related behavioural factors in four key WASH areas – hand washing, faeces handling and disposal, water treatment and storage, and menstrual blood management. The programme then developed and tested improved practices in the households in Kampala and Kamuli districts, from which it developed tools and manuals for home-based care workers.

In May 2009, USAID/HIP and Plan/Uganda conducted a pilot training of home-based care providers from organizations that provide home-based care services. A training of master trainers took place in September 2009 to replicate trainings in each participating organization. Organizations will also receive technical assistance in planning and implementing integration activities. Training materials and guides are on the USAID/HIP web site (http://www.hip.watsan.net).

To enrich these measures, and to ensure their sustainability and uptake in the sector, HIP initiated a subgroup on Sanitation & Hygiene Integration in HIV/AIDS, in partnership with the Uganda Water and Sanitation Network, under the National Sanitation Working Group.

For more information, contact Elizabeth Younger, eyounger@aed.org.

5.3.9 Vietnam – integration of safe water systems and health communications in care and support services

PSI is working closely with CARE and community-based organization partners to improve and increase access among PLHIV, and orphans and vulnerable children to the SafeWat safe water system and to behaviour change communications.[1] The aim is to promote correct and consistent household water treatment and good hygiene practices among PLHIV, orphans and vulnerable children, and their affected households. Safe water and hygiene promotion activities are integrated into existing care and support services in provinces particularly affected by cholera, to reduce the incidence of diarrhoeal diseases among immunocompromised and otherwise vulnerable populations in Hanoi, Ho Chi Minh City, Quang Ninh, Can Tho and An Giang.

Specific activities

The project integrates SafeWat promotion and hygiene awareness into existing community outreach events with PLHIV, orphans and vulnerable children, and their families. This has increased the acceptability of targeted communication messages. The project has trained local community-based organization partners on the links between unsafe drinking water, health and recommended good hygiene practices. Nutrition training in the south and north provinces also included this WASH component. Continuing interpersonal communication sessions and product demonstrations have built self-efficacy among potential users, demonstrated the effectiveness of SafeWat and encouraged the initial trial of SafeWat. Findings from programme implementation monitoring and research into current safe water practices, user experiences and reasons why some users lapsed will inform the phase 2 design of the project.

---

[1] http://www.changemakers.com/en-us/node/7055

Results

- Since the project launched in August 2008, over 20 000 SafeWat bottles have been distributed to HIV-affected households. Over 18 000 leaflets, posters and flipcharts have been distributed through 23 local partner organizations.

- Programme activities reached over 18 000 people: PLHIV (4875), orphans and vulnerable children (4025), and family members or caregivers (9315).

For more information, contact Cecilia Kwak, ckwak@psi.org.

5.4   Conclusion

This is the first time that information on integrating WASH and HIV has been systematically brought together to assist country-level programming. In the three years since USAID/HIP began exploring this topic, many new activities that integrate WASH and HIV have evolved, and are being documented and shared. This publication was developed to accelerate the process so that WASH becomes a routine part of HIV prevention and care, and HIV considerations are automatically included in water and sanitation programmes around the world.

WASH is essential to living a dignified life. Yet the knowledge and tools that make improved WASH practices possible are beyond the means of many people, especially those affected by HIV. In response to this reality, this document represents a call to action for all WASH and HIV practitioners. It asks them to work diligently to integrate these important health considerations and to document, share and promote their experiences widely to improve people's lives.

Bibliography and further reading

Ansari SA, Farrah SR, Chaudhry GR (1992). Presence of human immunodeficiency virus nucleic acids in wastewater and their detection by polymerase chain reaction. *Applied and Environmental Microbiology,* 58(12):3984–3990.

Aragon TJ et al.(2003). Endemic cryptosporidiosis and exposure to municipal tap water in persons with acquired immunodeficiency syndrome (AIDS): a case-control study. *BMC Public Health,* 6(32):2.

Aronson T et al. (1999). Comparison of large restriction fragments of *Mycobacterium avium* isolates recovered from AIDS and non-AIDS patients with those of isolates from potable water. *Journal of Clinical Microbiology,* 37(4):1008–1012.

Ashton P, Ramasar V (2002). Water and HIV/AIDS: some strategic considerations in Southern Africa. In: Turton A, Henwood R, eds. *Hydropolitics in the developing world: a southern African perspective.* Pretoria, African Water Issues Research Unit, 217–238(http://www.internationalwaterlaw.org/bibliography/articles/hydropolitics-s-africa.html).

Badri M et al. (2006). When to initiate highly active antiretroviral therapy in sub-Saharan Africa? A South African cost-effectiveness study. *Antiviral Therapy,* 11(1):63–72.

Bland RM et al. (2007). Infant feeding counselling for HIV-infected and uninfected women: appropriateness of choice and practice. *Bulletin of the World Health Organization,* 85(4):289–296.

Brink AK et al. (2002). Diarrhea,CD4 counts and enteric infections in a community-based cohort of HIV-infected adults in Uganda. *Journal of Infection,* 45:99–106.

Bushen OY et al. (2004). Diarrhea and reduced levels of antiretroviral drugs: improvement with glutamine or alanyl-glutamine in a randomized controlled trial in northeast Brazil. *Clinical Infectious Diseases,* 38(12):1764–1770.

CDC (1999). *HIV and its transmission.* Atlanta, GA, United States Centers for Disease Control and Prevention (http://www.cdc.gov/hiv/resources/factsheets/PDF/transmission.pdf).

CDC (2007a). *What you need to know about HIV and AIDS.* Altanta, GA, United States Centers for Disease Control and Prevention (http://www.cdc.gov/hiv/resources/brochures/careathome/care3.htm).

CDC (2007b). *What women can do*. Altanta, GA, United States Centers for Disease Control and Prevention (http://www.cdc.gov/hiv/topics/perinatal/protection.htm).

Chandler R, Decker C, Nziyige B (2004). *Estimating the cost of providing home-based care for HIV/AIDS in Rwanda*. Health Systems 20/20 (http://www.healthsystems2020.org/content/resource/detail/1454).

Clasen T et al. (2007). Interventions to improve water quality for preventing diarrhoea: systematic review and meta-analysis. *British Medical Journal*, 334(7597):782.

Colebunders R et al. (1987). Persistent diarrhea, strongly associated with HIV infection in Kinshasa, Zaire. *American Journal of Gastroenterology*, 82:859–864.

Colton T et al. (2006). *Community home-based care for people and communities affected by HIV/AIDS. A handbook for community health workers.* Watertown, MA, Pathfinder International (http://www.pathfind.org/site/DocServer/CHBC_HB_Complete.pdf?docID= 7961).

Colton T et al. (2006). Community home-based care for people and communities affected by HIV/AIDS. A comprehensive training course for community health workers: trainer's guide. Watertown, MA, Pathfinder International (http://www.pathfind.org/site/DocServer/CHBC_Trainer_s_Guide_Complet e.pdf?docID=8001).

Crump J et al. (2005). Household based treatment of drinking water with flocculant-disinfectant for preventing diarrhoea in areas with turbid source water in rural western Kenya: cluster randomised controlled trial. *British Medical Journal*, 331:478.

Curtis V, Cairncross S (2003). Effect of washing hands with soap on diarrhoea risk in the community: a systematic review. *Lancet Infectious Diseases*, 3(5):275–281.

DCP2 (Disease Control Priorities Project) (2006). *Disease control priorities in developing countries,* 2nd ed. New York, Oxford University Press (http://dcp2.org/pubs/DCP).

Doherty T et al. (2007). Effectiveness of the WHO/UNICEF guidelines on infant feeding for HIV-positive women: results from a prospective cohort study in South Africa. *Journal of Acquired Immune Deficiency Syndromes,* 21(13):1791–1797.

Family Health International (2004). *Module 4: monitoring and evaluating community home-based care programs*. Research Triangle Park, NC, Family Health International (http://www.fhi.org/NR/rdonlyres/ehz3d4ozmhbvbqijpcehueub57rj222dojjm 6nvyodu4ljdambpht2ipj5mxelce7w4ctj3eyyl5dc/Mod04.pdf).

Fewtrell L et al. (2005). Water, sanitation, and hygiene interventions to reduce diarrhoea in less developed countries: a systematic review and meta-analysis. *Lancet Infectious Diseases,* 5(1):42–52.

Fox S et al. (2002). Integrated community-based home care (ICHC) in South Africa: a review of the model implemented by the Hospice Association of South Africa. Cape Town, South Africa, POLICY Project (http://www.cadre.org.za/node/125).

Franks T, Cleaver F (2002). People, livelihoods and decision-making in catchment management: a case study from Tanzania. *Waterlines*, 20(3):7–10.

Goldie SJ et al. (2006). Cost-effectiveness of HIV treatment in resource-poor settings – the case of Côte d'Ivoire. *New England Journal of Medicine,* 355(11):1141–1153.

Grant AD, Djomand G, De Cock KM (1997). Natural history and spectrum of disease in adults with HIV/AIDS in Africa. *Journal of Acquired Immune Deficiency Syndromes*, 11(Suppl. B):S43–S54.

Harris J et al. (2009). Effect of a point-of-use water treatment and safe water storage intervention on diarrhea in infants of HIV-infected mothers. *Journal of Infectious Diseases*, 200(8):1186–1193.

Hillbrunner C (2007). Workshop on integration of water, sanitation and hygiene into HIV/AIDS home-based care strategies: background paper. Baltimore, MD, Catholic Relief Services.

Hillebrand-Haverkort ME et al. (1999). Generalized *Mycobacterium genavense* infection in HIV-infected patients: detection of the mycobacterium in hospital tap water. *Scandinavian Journal of Infectious Diseases,* 31(1):63–68.

HIP (2006). *Integrating hygiene improvement into HIV/AIDS programming to reduce diarrhea morbidity.* Washington DC, United States Agency for International Development (http://www.hip.watsan.net/content/download/1528/7298/file/HIP%20HI%20and%20HIV-AIDS%20integration8-06.pdf).

HIP (2007). Analysis of research on the effects of improved water, sanitation, and hygiene on the health of people living with HIV and AIDS and programmatic implications. Washington DC, United States Agency for International Development.

HIP (2008). *Programming water, sanitation, and hygiene (WASH) activities in U.S. government operational plans: a toolkit for FY2010 planning.* Washington, DC, United States Agency for International Development (http://www.hip.watsan.net/page/2709).

HIP (2008). *Programming guidance for integrating water, sanitation, and hygiene improvement into HIV/AIDS programs.* Washington DC, United States Agency for International Development.

Hsi N, Musau S, Chanfreau C (2005). *HIV/AIDS home-based care costing guidelines.* Bethesda, MD, PHRplus (http://pdf.usaid.gov/pdf_docs/PNADE226.pdf).

Huang DB, Zhou J (2007). Effect of intensive handwashing in the prevention of diarrhaeal illness among patients with AIDS: a randomized controlled study. *Journal of Medical Microbiology,* 56(5):659–663.

IASC (2004). *IASC Guidelines for HIV/AIDS interventions in emergency settings.* Geneva, World Health Organization (http://www.who.int/3by5/publications/documents/en/iasc_guidelines.pdf).

IRC (2006). *Girl-friendly toilets for school girls: helping adolescent girls.* Delft, IRC International Water and Sanitation Centre (http://www.schools.watsan.net/page/319).

IRC (2007a). *HIV/AIDS: making the links with WASH.* Delft, IRC International Water and Sanitation Centre (http://www.irc.nl/page/32435).

IRC (2007b). HIV/AIDS: caring for HIV-infected people in South Africa requires love, patience and 200 liters of water per day. *SOURCE Newsletter, May* 200, Delft, IRC International Water and Sanitation Centre (http://www.irc.nl/page/36137).

Joloba M et al. (2000). Determination of drug susceptibility and DNA fingerprint patterns of clinical isolates of *Mycobacterium tuberculosis* from Kampala, Uganda. *East African Medical Journal,* 77(2):111–115.

Jones H, Reed B (2005). *Water and sanitation for disabled people and other vulnerable groups: designing services to improve accessibility.* Leicestershire, UK, Water, Engineering and Development Centre (WEDC), Loughborough University.

Kamminga E, Wegelin-Schuringa M (2005). *HIV/AIDS and water, sanitation and hygiene: thematic overview paper.* Delft, IRC International Water and Sanitation Centre (http://www.irc.nl/page/3462).

Kangamba M et al. (2006). *Water and sanitation assessment of home-based care clients in Zambia.* Baltimore, MD, Catholic Relief Services (http://pdf.usaid.gov/pdf_docs/PNADJ423.pdf).

Kaplan JE et al. (1996). Preventing opportunistic infections in human immunodeficiency virus-infected persons: implications for the developing world. *American Journal of Tropical Medicine and Hygiene,* 55:1–11.

Kenya National AIDS/STD Control Programme (2002). *National home-based care programme and service guidelines.* Nairobi, Ministry of Health.

Kgalushi R, Smits S, Eales K (2004). People living with HIV/AIDS in a context of rural poverty: the importance of water and sanitation services and hygiene education. A case study from Bolobedu (Limpopo Province, South Africa). Johannesburg, South Africa, The Mvula Trust and Delft, IRC International Water and Sanitation Centre (http://www.irc.nl/content/download/11414/167794/file/Case_study_Limpop o_South_Af.pdf).

Kiongo JM (2005). The Millennium Development Goal on poverty and the links with water supply, sanitation, hygiene and HIV/AIDS: a case study from Kenya. Delft, IRC International Water and Sanitation Centre (http://www.irc.nl/page/16127).

Kirk J, Sommer M (2005). Menstruation and body awareness: critical issues for girls' education. *EQUALS*, 15:4–5 (http://www.oxfam.org.uk/what_we_do/issues/education/downloads/equals 15.pdf).

Lamptey PR, Gayle HD, eds (2001). *HIV/AIDS prevention care resource-constrained settings: a handbook for the design and management of programs.* Research Triangle Park, NC, Family Health International (http://www.fhi.org/NR/rdonlyres/eh7tyyfcpwmy6w3okmfxspm3cyenzp55ja ooz3omemjlghh3w4sn2dnybkbhw3sq4cegcvefivihmm/HIVAIDSPrevention Care1enhv.pdf).

Lantana CF (2003). Studies of food hygiene and diarrhoeal disease. *International Journal of Environmental Health Research*, 13(Suppl. 1):S175–S183.

Laurent P (2005). *Household drinking water systems and their impact on people with weakened immunity.* Geneva, World Health Organization (http://www.who.int/household_water/research/HWTS_impacts_on_weake ned_immunity.pdf).

Lockwood K et al. (2006). *Water and sanitation assessment of home-based care clients in Malawi.* Baltimore, MD, Catholic Relief Services (http://pdf.usaid.gov/pdf_docs/PNADJ422.pdf).

Luby SP et al. (2004). Effect of intensive handwashing promotion on childhood diarrhea in high-risk communities in Pakistan: a randomized controlled trial. *Journal of the American Medical Association,* 291(21):2547–2554.

Luby SP et al. (2005). Effect of handwashing on child health: a randomised controlled trial. *The Lancet*, 366:225–233.

Lule J et al. (2005). Effect of home-based water chlorination and safe storage on diarrhea among persons with human immunodeficiency virus in Uganda. *American Journal of Tropical Medicine and Hygiene*, 73(5):926–933.

Ma L et al. (2009). Efficacy of protocols for cleaning and disinfecting infant feeding bottles in less developed communities. *American Journal of Tropical Medicine and Hygiene*, 81(1):132–139.

Magrath P, Tesfu M (2006). *Meeting the needs for water and sanitation of people living with HIV/AIDS in Addis Ababa, Ethiopia*. Addis Ababa, WaterAid Ethiopia (http://www.wateraid.org/documents/plugin_documents/hivaids_equal_acc ess_for_all_no._6_april_2006.pdf).

Malawi Gender and Community Services (2003). *National policy on orphans and other vulnerable children*. Lilongwe, Malawi Ministry of Gender and Community Services.

Malawi Ministry of Health (2005). *National community home based care policy and guidelines*. Lilongwe, Malawi Ministry of Health.

Malawi National AIDS Commission. (2003). *Malawi national HIV/AIDS policy: a call for renewed action*. Lilongwe, National AIDS Commission (http://www.who.int/hiv/Malawi-HIVAIDS-Policy.pdf).

Mata L (1988). Diarrhoea and AIDS. *Dialogue Diarrhoea*, (35):3.

Meier A et al. (2006). Independent association of hygiene, socioeconomic status, and circumcision with reduced risk of HIV infection among Kenyan men. *Journal of Acquired Immune Deficiency Syndromes*, 43(1):117–118.

Mermin J et al. (2005). Developing an evidence-based, preventive care package for persons with HIV in Africa. *Tropical Medicine and International Health*, 10(10):961–970.

Millennium Water Alliance. *Quality of life: exploring the links between living with HIV/AIDS and safe water and sanitation*. (http://www.mwawater.org/mwadatabase/Briefs/tabid/61/Default.aspx).

Mohammed N, Gikonyo J (2005). Operational challenges: community home based care (CHBC) for PLWHA in multi-country HIV/AIDS programs (MAP) for sub-Saharan Africa. Washington DC, World Bank (http://www.worldbank.org/afr/wps/wp88.pdf).

Molose V, Potter A, Mvula Trust (2007). Understanding the links between AIDS, water and sanitation and hygiene: experiences from Jeppe's Reef. Nkomazi LM Mpumalanga.

Moore BE (1993). Survival of human immunodeficiency virus (HIV), HIV-infected lymphocytes, and poliovirus in water. *Applied and Environmental Microbiology*, 59(5):1437–1443.

Morris SS, Black RE, Tomaskovic L (2003). Predicting the distribution of under-five deaths by cause in countries without adequate vital registration systems. *International Journal of Epidemiology*, 32:1041–1051.

Ngwenya BN, Kgathi DL (2006). HIV/AIDS and access to water: a case study of home-based care in Ngamiland, Botswana. *Physics and Chemistry of the Earth*, 31:669–680.

Obi CL et al. (2006). The interesting cross-paths of HIV/AIDS and water in southern Africa with special reference to South Africa. *Water SA*, 32(3):323–344. (http://www.wrc.org.za/Pages/DisplayItem.aspx?ItemID=5292&FromURL=%2fPages%2fKH_WaterSA.aspx%3fdt%3d5%26ms%3d56%253b).

Onadeko MO, Joynson DH, Payne RA (1992). The prevalence of *Toxoplasma* infection among pregnant women in Ibadan, Nigeria. *Journal of Tropical Medicine and Hygiene*, 95(2):143–145.

O'Reilly CE et al. (2008). The impact of a school-based safe water and hygiene programme on knowledge and practices of students and their parents: Nyanza Province, western Kenya. *Epidemiology and Infection,* 136:80–91.

Parker AA et al. (2006). Sustained high levels of stored drinking water treatment and retention of hand-washing knowledge in rural Kenyan households following a clinic-based intervention. *Epidemiology and Infection*, 134(5):1029–1036.

Potgieter N, Koekemoer R, JagalsP (2007). A pilot assessment of water, sanitation, hygiene and home-based care services for people living with HIV/AIDS in rural and peri-urban communities in South Africa. *Water Science & Technology*, 56(5):125–131.

Potter A, Clacherty A (2007). Water services and HIV/AIDS. Water, sanitation and health and hygiene education in the context of HIV/AIDS: a guide for local government councillors and officials responsible for water, sanitation and municipal health services. Pretoria, South Africa, Water Research Commission.

QUEST (n.d.) *Improving the management of sexual maturation in primary schools in Kenya, Uganda and Zimbabwe: a concept paper.* Rockefeller Foundation, Quality Education for Social Transformation, (http://www.questafrica.org/GrowingUp.aspx).

Reichelderfer PS et al. (2000). Effect of menstrual cycle on HIV-1 levels in the peripheral blood and genital tract. *Journal of Acquired Immune Deficiency Syndromes*, 14(14):2101–2107.

SA Department of Health (2001). *National guideline on home-based care and community-based care.* South African Department of Health (http://www.capegateway.gov.za/xho/publications/guidelines_manuals_and_instructions/N/3654).

Schuler N (2005). *Lessons and experiences from Mainstreaming HIV/AIDS into urban/water (AFTU1 & 2) projects.* Washington DC, World Bank (http://www-wds.worldbank.org/external/default/main?pagePK=64193027&piPK=64187937&theSitePK=523679&menuPK=64187510&searchMenuPK=64187283&siteName=WDS&entityID=000012009_20051019135310).

Senefeld S, Powell A (2009). *Integration of water, sanitation and hygiene into HIV programs: lessons from Malawi*. Baltimore, MD, Catholic Relief Services (http://www.crsprogramquality.org/2009/11/integrating-water-sanitation-hygiene-hiv-programs).

Shahid NS et al. (1996). Hand washing with soap reduces diarrhoea and spread of bacterial pathogens in a Bangladesh village. *Journal of Diarrhoeal Disease Research*, 14(2):85–89.

Short RV (2006). New ways of preventing HIV infection: thinking simply, simply thinking. *Philosophical Transactions of the Royal Society of London B (Biological Sciences)*, 361(1469):811–820.

Shrestha RK et al. (2006). Cost-effectiveness of home-based chlorination and safe water storage in reducing diarrhea among HIV-affected households in rural Uganda. *American Journal of Tropical Medicine and Hygiene*, 74(5):884–890.

Sobsey M (2002). *Managing water in the home: accelerated health gains from improved water supply*. Geneva, World Health Organization, (WHO/SDE/WSH/02.07) (http://www.who.int/water_sanitation_health/dwq/wsh0207/en).

Sorvillo F et al. (1994). Municipal drinking water and cryptosporidiosis among persons with AIDS in Los Angeles County. *Epidemiology and Infection*, 113(2):313–320.

Tanzania Ministry of Health (2005). *Guidelines for home based care services*. Dar Es Salaam, Ministry of Health (http://www.nacp.go.tz/modules/doc_sm/admin/docs/Guidelines%20for%20HBC%20Services%20Feb-2005_1.pdf).

Taylor RH et al. (2000). Chlorine, chloramine, chlorine dioxide, and ozone susceptibility of *Mycobacterium avium*. *Applied and Environmental Microbiology*, 66(4):1702–1705.

Thior I et al. (2006). Breastfeeding plus infant zidovudine prophylaxis for 6 months vs formula feeding plus infant zidovudine for 1 month to reduce mother-to-child HIV transmission in Botswana. A randomized trial: the Mashi study. *Journal of the American Medical Association*, 296(7):794–805.

UN-HABITAT (2007). *HIV/AIDS checklist for water and sanitation projects*. Nairobi, United Nations Human Settlements Programme (http://www.unhabitat.org/pmss/getPage.asp?page=bookView&book=2068).

UNICEF (2001). *Teacher's guide for the integrated water, sanitation and hygiene education, and HIV/AIDS for grades 1 to 7*. Lusaka, Zambia, United Nations Children's Fund (http://www.schoolsanitation.org/Resources/Readings/Zambia_teachersguide%5B1%5D.pdf).

UNICEF (2002a). *HIV and infant feeding: a UNICEF fact sheet*. New York, United Nations Children's Fund.

UNICEF (2002b). *Maternal to child transmission of HIV: a UNICEF fact sheet*. New York, United Nations Children's Fund.

UNICEF & IRC (2005). Water, sanitation and hygiene education for schools roundtable meeting. Roundtable proceedings and framework for action. Meeting Oxford, 24–26 January 2005. The Hague, The Netherlands, United Nations Children's Fund and IRC International Water and Sanitation Centre (http://www.irc.nl/page/25321).

UN-Water (2008). *Sanitation: a wise investment for health, dignity, and development*. United Nations Water. (http://esa.un.org/iys/docs/IYS%20Advocacy%20kit%20ENGLISH/Key%20 messages%20booklet.pdf).

USAID (2004). *Environmental health: technical and program background*. Bureau for Global Health, Office of Health, Infectious Diseases, and Nutrition. Washington, DC, United States Agency for International Development (http://www.usaid.gov/our_work/global_health/home/News/ehaad.pdf).

van der Hoek L et al. (1995). Isolation of human immunodeficiency virus type 1 (HIV-1) RNA from feces by a simple method and difference between HIV-1 subpopulations in feces and serum. *Journal of Clinical Microbiology*, 33(3):581–588.

Voss JG, Sukati NA, Seboni NM (2007). Symptom burden of fatigue in men and women living with HIV/AIDS in Southern Africa. *Journal of the Association of Nurses in AIDS Care*, 18(4):22–31.

Walensky RP et al. (2007). HIV drug resistance surveillance for prioritizing treatment in resource-limited settings. *Journal of Acquired Immune Deficiency Syndromes*, 21(8):973–982.

WaterAid (2006). Assessment of the adequacy of water, sanitation and hygiene facilities in resource-poor areas of Nigeria in relation to the needs of vulnerable people. Abuja, Nigeria:WaterAid Nigeria.

WaterAid (2009). *Making the links: mapping the relationship between water, hygiene and sanitation, and HIV/AIDS*: a joint think-piece by WaterAid Ethiopia and Progynist. London, WaterAid (http://www.wateraid.org/documents/makinglinks.pdf).

WEF (2000). *Can AIDS be transmitted by biosolids?* WEF/U.S. EPA biosolids fact sheet. Alexandria, VA, Water Environment Federation (http://www.biosolids.org/docs/AIDS.pdf).

Wegelin-Schuringa M, Kamminga E (2006). Water and sanitation in the context of HIV/AIDS – the right of access in resource-poor countries. *Health and Human Rights,* 9(1):153–172.

Wegelin-Schuringa M, Kamminga E, de Graaf S (2003). HIV/AIDS and its implications for the water and sanitation sector. In: Harvey P, ed. *Towards the Millenium Development* Goals, 29th International Conference, Abuja, Nigeria: WEDC (http://wedc.lboro.ac.uk/knowledge/know).

Wegelin-Schuringa M, Tiendrebeogo G, eds. (2004). Techniques and practices for local responses to HIV/AIDS. Part 1: techniques. Part 2: practices. Amsterdam, KIT Publishers and Geneva, UNAIDS.

WELL Project (2004a). *WELL Briefing Note: The HIV/AIDS Millennium Development Goal – What water, sanitation and hygiene can do.* London, WELL Project (http://www.lboro.ac.uk/well/resources/Publications/Briefing%20Notes/BN%20HIV%20AIDS.htm).

WELL Project (2004b). *The HIV/AIDS Millennium Development Goal: HIV/AIDS and water supply, sanitation and hygiene in Southern Africa.* London, WELL Project (http://www.lboro.ac.uk/well/resources/Publications/Briefing%20Notes/WELL%20HIV%20Poster%20Southern%20Africa%20NC.pdf).

WHO (2000). *Home-based long-term care: report of a WHO study group.* Geneva, World Health Organization (http://whqlibdoc.who.int/trs/WHO_TRS_898.pdf).

WHO (2002a). *Community home-based care in resource-limited settings: a framework for action.* Geneva, World Health Organization (http://www.who.int/chp/knowledge/publications/comm_home_based_care.pdf).

WHO (2002b). *Living well with HIV/AIDS: a manual on nutritional care and support for people living with HIV/AIDS.* Rome, Food and Agriculture Organization (http://www.fao.org/docrep/005/y4168e/y4168e00.HTM).

WHO (2003). *Emerging issues in water and infectious disease.* Geneva, World Health Organization (http://www.who.int/water_sanitation_health/emerging/emerging.pdf).

WHO (2006). *Guidelines for drinking water quality.* Geneva, World Health Organization (http://www.who.int/water_sanitation_health/dwq/gdwq3rev/en/index.html).

WHO (2007a). *Combating waterborne disease at the household level.* Geneva, World Health Organization (http://www.who.int/water_sanitation_health/publications/combating_disease/en/index.html).

WHO (2007b). Infection prevention and control of epidemic- and pandemic- prone acute respiratory diseases in health care - WHO interim guidelines. Geneva, World Health Organization (http://www.who.int/csr/bioriskreduction/infection_control/publications/en/in dex.html).

WHO (2008). *Essential environmental health standards in health care.* Geneva, World Health Organization (http://www.who.int/water_sanitation_health/hygiene/settings/ehs_hc/en/in dex.html).

WHO (2009a). *Five keys to safer food manual.* Geneva, World Health Organization. (http://www.who.int/foodsafety/publications/consumer/manual_keys.pdf).

WHO (2009b). *Water, Sanitation and Hygiene Standards for Schools in Low-cost Settings.* Geneva, World Health Organization. (http://www.who.int/water_sanitation_health/publications/wsh_standards_s chool/en/index.html).

WHO (2009c). *WHO Guidelines on Hand Hygiene in Health Care.* Geneva, World Health Organization. (http://whqlibdoc.who.int/publications/2009/9789241597906_eng.pdf).

WHO/PAHO (2009). *Sterilization manual for health centres.* Washington, Pan American Health Organization / World Health Organization.

WHO (2010). A summary of evidence for the revised WHO principles and recommendations on HIV and infant feeding. Geneva, World Health Organization.

Wijk van C (2003). *WELL Factsheet: HIV/AIDS and water supply, sanitation and hygiene.* London, WELL Project (http://www.lboro.ac.uk/well/resources/fact-sheets/fact-sheets-htm/hiv-aids.htm).

WSP (2007). Water, sanitation, and hygiene for people living with HIV and AIDS. Washington DC, Water and Sanitation Program (http://www-wds.worldbank.org/servlet/main?menuPK=64187510&pagePK=64193027 &piPK=64187937&theSitePK=523679&entityID=000310607_20071003160 417).

WSSCC, Water, Engineering and Development Centre (2004). *For her it's the big issue: putting women at the centre of water supply, sanitation and hygiene.* Water, Sanitation and Hygiene Evidence Report. Geneva, Water Supply and Sanitation Collaborative Council.

Zambia National Food and Nutrition Commission (2004). *Nutrition guidelines for care and support of people living with HIV/AIDS.* Lusaka, National Food and Nutrition Commission.

Zimbabwe (2004). *Zimbabwe water and sanitation sector HIV/AIDS response: programme, strategies and guidelines.* Zimbabwe: National Action Committee, Government of Zimbabwe, United Nations Children's Fund (http://www.sarpn.org.za/documents/d0001030/Water_HIV_AIDS_Response_Guidelines_June2003.pdf).

Zimbabwe Ministry of Health and Child Welfare (2004). *National community home-based standards.* Harare, Ministry of Health.

Annexes

Annex 1 Process development and affiliations of all group members

A1.1 Process for developing the WASH–HIV integration guideline

This publication was developed over the past three years, drawing on documents and input from experts and field-based projects. In 2007, Dr Kate Tulenko, then of the World Bank, conducted a review of the literature on WASH and HIV with the specific purpose of identifying gaps in the evidence base and suggesting next steps for research in this area of integration. The HIP (tasked through its contract mandate to integrate WASH into 'other' technical areas to achieve WASH at scale) then adapted and updated this focused literature review to a more programmatic context and audience, clearly and simply reviewing the evidence base. From this, the project suggested evidence-based programming options for strengthening WASH in HIV programmes. Additional documents included in the expanded literature review were identified and reviewed by Dan Campbell, Web Manager for Environmental Health at USAID, who oversees a well-established clearinghouse and referral center for WASH-related literature and tools.

Concurrent to this process, WHO, with funding from USAID, called for proposals from countries to assess the 'Adequacy of water, sanitation and hygiene in relation to home-based care strategies for people living with HIV/AIDS'. The assessments were carried out in Nigeria, Malawi, Zambia, China, South Africa and Vietnam. The findings from the assessments varied according to the context of the country, but similar themes emerged from the assessments, including a need to integrate water, sanitation and hygiene more closely into home-based care programmes.

The WHO/Malawi assessment was carried out by CRS from January to July 2006 and examined water, sanitation and hygiene arrangements in two rural and two urban poor community settings in Malawi. This was done to determine their adequacy with respect to home-based care policies and people living with HIV and AIDS. This assessment was the first known work of its kind to examine the current water and sanitation situation of home-based care clients in Malawi. Relevant national and local level policies and strategies, shortfalls in implementation, and roles and responsibilities of all stakeholders were also investigated. The findings from the assessment verified that WASH is indeed an intervention area requiring additional attention within home-based care programming. One recommendation emerging from the Malawi assessment was the need to convene a national workshop of key stakeholders in key sectors of HIV and WASH to come to a consensus on how to move the integration agenda forward.

With the remaining USAID funding, WHO and USAID cosponsored a workshop in Malawi in late 2007 as a concrete step in advancing the integration of HIV/AIDS and WASH programming in the country. The updated HIP literature review with programming guidance ('Analysis of research on the effects of improved water, sanitation and hygiene on the health of people living with HIV/AIDS and programmatic implications') was used as a background paper for this conference. This paper, assessment of country policies and programmatic implications was vetted by over 50 participants from different NGOs, international technical specialists, donor agencies and government departments attending the workshop.

Concurrently, USAID/HIP developed specific programming guidance to guide the PEPFAR initiative in different countries by including WASH when developing their country operational plans. As a result, water, sanitation and hygiene programming is now included in at least 15 PEPFAR country plans.

Over a three year period, growing interest in the area of integration of WASH into HIV programmes received increased attention and increased funding. WHO and USAID in particular championed efforts to integrate WASH and HIV in a more concerted manner. USAID/HIP was part of a group of international and national organizations supporting pilot efforts to integrate WASH at the country policy and programming level. Specifically, USAID/HIP and other AED projects assisted efforts in Ethiopia, Uganda, Malawi, and now Tanzania and Kenya to integrate WASH into HIV.

In June 2008, WHO and USAID decided to write this practical document in response to requests from countries and programmes for concrete guidance on how to integrate WASH practices into HIV policies and programmes. Guidance, tools and experience from country-level applications, including the WHO/CRS work in Malawi, were incorporated into this final document currently under review within WHO. The authors started with the HIP-prepared Malawi background document and the USAID Country Operational Programming guidance, incorporating additional material to address the expanded mandate of this document under review – to provide programming guidance from policy to programme level for integrating WASH into HIV programmes. Where information was particularly scarce, the authors contacted researchers and experts who work or live in resource-poor contexts. The authors contacted many people working in different countries, primarily in Africa, to discover what is currently being done in WASH–HIV integration. The authors also canvassed the reviewers and potential reviewers for examples that were not based in Africa. These were limited, as the burden of the disease, as well as funding for care and support programmes, has been concentrated in Africa to date. The authors, with assistance from Lonna Shafritz, senior programme officer at AED, reviewed entire HIV policy documents from countries receiving PEPFAR assistance. This was an effort to include additional geographic representation from countries other than African nations, which led to government documents from other large countries, such as India. These documents were identified by researching web sites and through assistance from contacts working in these countries.

In July 2009, the document was then carefully reviewed by a host of independent reviewers (names and affiliations listed in section A1.2, below) with no direct affiliation to the authors, but with established expertise in the area of HIV or WASH (or both). Their expert comments were used to finalize the document. In September 2009, the updated version was shared for peer review with a larger number of international experts.

This document was driven by professionalism and passion for the subject area, using established research methods, and evidence and experience-base for all programming recommendations. The authors have no commercial interest nor other conflict of interest in seeing this document published.

A1.2 Affiliations of all group members

Name	Region/ country	Affiliation and specification	Area of expertise	Main involvement in the document
Renuka Bery	Washington, DC, USA	AED, with funding from USAID	Master of Public Health with expertise in water, sanitation and hygiene and communication	Author
Julia Rosenbaum	Washington, DC, USA	AED, with funding from USAID	Master of Science in Public Health with expertise in water, sanitation and hygiene; deputy director for HIP	Author
Julie Chitty	New Delhi, India	Consultant	Developed WASH–HIV programme in Uganda and WASH–HIV materials for US Government audience for AED	Wrote documents that were adapted for this publication; reviewed draft version
Yves Chartier	Geneva, Switzerland	WHO	Public health engineer; water and sanitation expertise	Conceptualized this document; provided input into draft version; reviewed final version
Merri Weinger	Washington, DC, USA	USAID	Programme manager for hygiene; water and sanitation expertise	Conceptualized this document; provided input into draft version; reviewed final version
Robert Quick	Atlanta, GA, USA	US Centers for Disease Control and Prevention	Medical epidemiologist; conducts research on diarrheal disease prevention	Provided input into draft version
Libertad Gonzalez	Nairobi, Kenya	Federation of the Red Cross	Communication within the WASH Unit	Provided input into draft version; shared resources
Foyeke Tolani	United Kingdom	Oxfam	WASH–HIV coordinator	Provided input into draft version
Ben Harvey	New York, USA	IRC	Water and sanitation expert	Provided input into draft version
Kate Tulenko	Washington, DC, USA	World Bank	Medical doctor and public health expert	Wrote a literature review on WASH and HIV that was

				adapted for this publication
Alana Potter	Delft, Netherlands	IRC	Hygiene and sanitation specialist; worked on WASH and HIV in South Africa	Provided input into draft version
Dennis Warner	Baltimore, MD, USA	CRS	WASH team leader	Reviewed final version
Antonia Powell	Malawi	CRS	Country director	Provided input into draft version
Eleonore Seumo	Washington, DC, USA	AED	WASH–HIV trainer	Wrote materials on WASH and HIV; provided input into draft version
Elizabeth Younger	Washington, DC, USA	The Manoff Group	Developed and managed WASH–HIV programme in Uganda	Provided input into draft version
Marie Coughlan	Connecticut, USA	Save the Children	Public health nurse and trainer	Developed initial HIP WASH–HIV training
Lonna Shafritz	Washington, DC, USA	AED	Public health background with expertise in HIV, WASH, communication	Reviewed country policies from PEPFAR countries; provided input into draft version
Anne Kerisel	Geneva, Switzerland	WHO consultant	Editor	Provided input into draft and final version
Sandra Callier	Washington, DC, USA	AED	Project director for HIP	Provided input into draft version
Orlando Hernandez	Washington, DC, USA	AED	Monitoring and evaluation advisor for HIP	Provided input into draft version
Patricia Mantey	Washington, DC, USA	AED	Knowledge management advisor, HIP	Provided input into draft version
Peter Maes	Belgium	Médecins Sans Frontières	Public health engineer; water and sanitation expertise	Provided input into draft version
Maryline Mulemba	France	Médecins Sans Frontières	Public health nurse with high expertise in HIV	Provided input into draft version
Shannon Senefield	Baltimore, MD, USA	CRS	Senior technical advisor for HIV and AIDS	Provided input into draft version

Nathalie van Meerbeeck	Belgium	Médecins Sans Frontières	Infection control advisor	Provided input into draft version
Dan Campbell	Washington, DC, USA	USAID	Web manager, Environmental Health	Identified and reviewed literature on WASH and HIV

AED, Academy for Educational Development; AIDS, acquired immune deficiency syndrome; CRS, Catholic Relief Services; HIP, Hygiene Improvement Project; HIV, human immunodeficiency virus; IRC, International Rescue Committee; PEPFAR, President's Emergency Plan for AIDS Relief; USAID, United States Agency for International Development; WASH, water, sanitation and hygiene; WHO, World Health Organization

A1.3 Information on the Manoff Group

The Manoff Group is a woman-owned small business based in Washington, DC that provides assistance in communication and behavior-centered programming to nutrition, health, environment, water and HIV/AIDS programmes. The firm has been at the forefront of social marketing development since it first applied commercial marketing techniques to social programmes in India in 1967. The Manoff Group has brought innovations in qualitative research methods, communication, media planning and materials development to programmes around the globe for 40 years. This focus continues in its work on counselling and negotiation skills, and developing tools to change behaviour and improve health outcomes. For additional information, see http://www.manoffgroup.com.

Annex 2   Why WASH?: examining the existing research

This annex incorporates and updates the 2006 literature review conducted by Kate Tulenko of Water and Sanitation Programme (WSP)/World Bank to document the evidence that links WASH and HIV (HIP, 2007).

A2.1 Water quality

Water quality, especially the absence of harmful bacteria, viruses and parasites, is known to be very important in preventing infection in people with full immune systems. A great irony exists in giving advanced, costly life-saving ART to PLHIV with a glass of water that could infect them with a life-threatening illness. It is important to maximize the effectiveness of these medicines by using safe water for ingesting them, since a side effect of many antiretroviral drugs is diarrhoea. Further, diarrhoeal illness in PLHIV can interfere with and compromise the absorption of these antiretroviral drugs and can even contribute to developing HIV strains that are resistant to antiviral agents (Bushen et al., 2004). Thus, safe drinking water becomes that much more compulsory as ART becomes more pervasive in the developing world.

A meta-analysis on interventions to improve microbial quality of water showed that improved water quality is generally effective in preventing diarrhoea (Clasen et al., 2007). In extrapolating these findings to PLHIV in low resources settings, the environment may be so contaminated that clean water will quickly become contaminated or that the pathogens will infect PLHIV through routes such as the oral–faecal route. In such settings, no amount of water treatment will likely have a measurable effect on PLHIV health. Nevertheless, evidence points towards improving water quality for better outcomes for PLHIV and for their affected families.

Two studies were found on water quality and PLHIV in developing countries. The most powerful is a random case control by Lule et al. of 392 households affected by HIV (including 509 PLHIV and their 1521 family members) randomized to use home chlorination, safe household water storage and basic hygiene education versus basic hygiene education alone (Lule et al., 2005). Intervention households reported 25% fewer diarrhoea episodes among PLHIV (a discrete case of diarrhoea having a specific beginning and end, and usually lasting from several days to several weeks) and 33% fewer days with diarrhoea. The health benefits were extended to household members. These benefits are important because compared to many targeted HIV and AIDS interventions that benefit only the target client, WASH services in general have the potential to improve the quality of life for the whole family and therefore increase their potential cost-effectiveness.

The Lule study found that the diarrhoea reduction for PLHIV did not extend to those who also consumed water outside the house. This group consisted mainly of people who worked outside the home and undoubtedly drank from contaminated sources outside the house. Lack of clean water should not be a barrier to employment outside the home since PLHIV need income. This evidence suggests the need to educate PLHIV on carrying adequate clean water supplies with them, or if possible, treating and storing clean water at their workplace.

Another interesting Lule study finding was that most households affected by HIV (60%) did not treat their water before the study and the most common treatment was boiling, a practice that is expensive (fuel), time-consuming (boiling and cooling), often improperly practiced (not boiling for adequate length of time) and is difficult to use to treat large volumes of water. Other studies (Kangamba et al., 2006; Lockwood et al., 2006; WSP, 2007) have yielded similar results. The WSP study in India found that while PLHIV adopted safer water and hygiene practices than the general population, water treatment was considered costly and time consuming.

A study of home-based care of end-stage PLHIV in Ngamiland, Botswana (two-stage stratified random sample survey) (Ngwengya & Kgathi, 2006), revealed that caregivers who experienced periodic water shortages due to equipment failure or temporary spikes in water costs reported using lower quality water sources, such as open wells, and surface water, such as rivers and lakes. The study did not measure adverse effects of this drop in water quality, but reinforces anecdotal evidence that as the financial or time cost of water rises, PLHIV must compromise on water quality and quantity. As household finances decrease, and time required for chores, such as water carrying increases, these data support the need for HIV/AIDS programmes to prioritize the value of safe water against other critical needs, such as housing quality, quality and quantity of food, access to medications, etc. Also, if the quality of the available water source declines, the need increases for PLHIV to use home-based water treatment and safe water handling.

Four studies were found on water quality for PLHIV in the developed world. For PLHIV in San Francisco, drinking tap water (as opposed to bottled water or treated tap water) was a risk for having cryptosporidiosis (Aragon et al., 2003). Tap water in developed countries was also found to be a source of atypical mycobacterial infections such as *Mycobacterium genavense* (Hillebrand-Haverkort et al., 1999) and *M. avium* (Aronson et al., 1999). The Aronson study found that water in hospitals was more likely to be contaminated (100%) than water in private homes (82%). This finding reinforces the need to clean water taps and handle water properly, especially in hospital settings where the risk of nosocomial infection is great.

Sorvillo et al. (1994) studied the effects of municipal water filtering on cryptosporidium infection in PLHIV. Until 1986, Los Angeles had two municipal water suppliers, one that used filters that would remove cryptosporidium spores and one that did not. PLHIV living in sections of the city provided with filtered tap water were 32% less likely to have cryptosporidiosis than those living in sections of the city provided with unfiltered tap water (4.2% compared to 6.2%).

Current water access and collection practice in the developing world virtually guarantees high contamination by the time water reaches the home. Rural and municipal water systems are notoriously undermaintained and too often contaminated at the source. This is further compounded by the perception that piped water is "safe", so few measures are taken to treat or protect drinking water.

A2.2 Water quantity

Water quantity is also a factor in caring for PLHIV, especially in late stage AIDS. The WSP Field Note on WASH and HIV in South Asia (June 2007) indicates that home-based care requires more than the 20 litres of water per person per day that is considered basic access, including an extra 1.5 litres of safe water for drinking with medicines such as ART. But, the study does not identify a specific amount of water required by HIV-affected households. A home-based care study in Ngamiland, Botswana (Ngwengya & Kgathi, 2006), revealed that caregivers who experienced periodic water shortages due to equipment failure or prohibitive costs reduced the frequency of bathing clients from twice daily to once daily or not at all. Although this study did not measure adverse effects of this change in bathing patterns, bathing and proper hygiene at end-stage has two clear benefits: preserving the dignity of PLHIV, and protecting caregivers and household members from infection with HIV or more likely, other disease-causing pathogens. For end-stage, bedridden PLHIV, caregivers reported requiring 20 to 80 additional litres of water per day, depending upon the severity of the client's symptoms, especially diarrhoea.

Molose and Potter (2007) interviewed PLHIV caregivers who reported that the average water needs for home-based care was 200 litres and included water for laundry, cooking, bathing and drinking. A large portion of the water, however, was also required for income generation schemes and food production. Anecdotal evidence suggested that hygiene improved based on water quantity, but the improvements were not quantified. The purpose of the effort was to document the voices and experiences of people living with and caring for people living with HIV/AIDS.

A2.2.1 Water access (cost, carrying distance, physical requirement at source)

No studies were found on the effect of water access on PLHIV, yet WSP has noted that lack of access has led to PLHIV using unsafe water. PLHIV experience periods of illness and relative weakness (Voss, Sukati & Seboni, 2007); during these periods they require close access to water and sanitation facilities. Studies have shown that those travelling great distances to collect water will reduce intake of water and use less safe water sources, and that those without easy access to latrines will often resort to open defecation methods (WSP, 2007). Increased access to water also assists PLHIV and their families to maintain kitchen gardens or engage in income generating activities that will help ensure food security, improved nutrition, and provide additional income for the household.

Women and girls in Africa and Asia walk, on average, six kilometres per day to collect water; collectively spending 40 billion hours every year fetching water (WSSCC, 2004). The WSP (2007) also observed that, on average, in India, women spend 2.2 hours per day fetching water, which translates into 150 million working days per year, or a cost of $208 million. Studies in Zambia (Kangamba et al., 2006) and Malawi (Lockwood et al., 2006) indicate that water access in rural areas is, on average, 400 metres away from the home, but facilities are poorly maintained. In urban areas, water is purchased but the cost can become prohibitive. WELL Briefing Note (Well Project 2004a) indicates that improved water supply eased domestic burdens and improved economic productivity. It is further noted that 10% more water used for domestic cleaning led to a 1.3% reduction in diarrhoea incidence in households with unknown HIV status.

Factors affecting access include the cost of water, the distance the water needs to be transported and the degree of physical effort needed to extract the water at the source (e.g. number of pounds of force needed to depress a pump handle and the number of times the handle needs to be pumped; the number of metres that a bucket needs to be pulled up a well).

Kamminga & Wegelin-Schuringa (2005) and others have also noted that PLHIV have less access to decisions being made in community-managed water systems, which can further limit access to water. The WSP study noted that PLHIV are highly marginalized in society due to stigma (WSP, 2007).

Several studies also mention the importance of water access in food security of HIV-affected households (Kgalushi, Smits & Eales, 2004; Kangamba et al., 2006; WELL Project, 2004b). In addition, many income generation activities such as beer making, food production and livestock rearing require accessible water (Kangamba et al., 2006), and these activities often ensure sufficient nutrition and the continued productive livelihoods for these households.

A2.3 Sanitation

Only one study found that improved sanitation enhances PLHIV health. The 2005 Lule study did not have sanitation as an intervention; however, researchers recorded the latrine access of all study participants and found that the presence of a latrine in the family compound was associated with fewer episodes of diarrhoea, fewer days with diarrhoea, and fewer days of work or school lost due to diarrhoea.

Since many waterborne pathogens that affect PLHIV, such as *M. avium*, are becoming increasingly resistant to water treatments such as chlorine, monochloramine, chlorine dioxide and ozone (Taylor et al., 2000), it is increasingly important to use sanitation to prevent the faecal contamination of drinking water.

Studies have revealed that in developing country settings, pathogens that affect PLHIV are generally the same as those that affect people with full immune systems, although the concentrations may be different (Lule et al., 2005). This is significant for two reasons: 1) if diarrhoea in PLHIV is mainly caused by infectious agents already present in the environment and the body, then improved WASH may not protect PLHIV and 2) if the diarrhoea of PLHIV is more highly concentrated and therefore more infectious than that of HIV negative people, then WASH efforts are critical to prevent further transmission of diarrhoea-causing pathogens in both PLHIV and other household members.

Kangamba et al. (2006) and Lockwood et al. (2006) found in Zambia and Malawi, respectively, that most home-based care clients had a latrine, but in many cases lack of water rendered these (flush) latrines unusable. Further, at least 20% of the latrines in both studies were poorly maintained, with faecal matter evident around them indicating prime transmission sites for waterborne pathogens. Barriers to improved sanitation were evident in both countries: inhospitable soils often led to latrine collapse; cultural beliefs prevented use; and cost, lack of donor interest and fewer adult male-headed households prevented new latrine construction. Further, in HIV-affected households, the available and diminishing resources were diverted to purchase food, medicine and, in some cases, water.

A2.3.1 Risks associated with sanitation and faeces

Faeces itself presents little risk of HIV infection, though great risk of transmitting diarrhoea-causing pathogens exists. HIV has never been isolated in urine or faeces (WEF, 2000), and international guidelines all rate the risk of HIV infection from faeces itself to be low to none (CDC, 2007a).

However, the faeces of end-stage PLHIV is likely to have increased amounts of blood and white blood cells carrying the HIV virus and the late-stage

PLHIV is more likely to have other infections that could affect household members.

Evaluating the risk of HIV transmission through faeces is highly contextual and guidelines encourage use of general precautions (gloves) when handling faeces or soiled clothing, and bed sheets. Whether this recommendation is feasible in a resource-poor household environment is questionable, particularly in light of the relatively low risk of HIV transmission. Several studies indicate that HIV, a very unstable virus, loses its infectivity soon after leaving the body. HIV is also rapidly inactivated by heat or the presence of a hostile environment, such as water or urine. Research also shows that the composition of faeces and urine quickly diminish the infectivity of any HIV virus present (Moore, 1993; WEF, 2000).

One study (Moore, 1993) showed that HIV-infected blood introduced into dechlorinated tap water had no detectable HIV virus after five minutes. Other scientists have placed concentrated HIV virus in faeces, wastewater and biosolids to study its survival. These studies have determined that urine and faeces inactivate the virus within one hour and in wastewater, the viral infectivity was gone within 48 hours (WEF, 2000), even at high concentrations that far exceed what would normally be found in wastewater.

Nonetheless, other infectious agents that cause diarrhoea are easily transmitted to caregivers and other household members unless faecal matter is cleared away quickly and thoroughly with water and a cleaning agent. This is discussed further in the hand-washing section, below.

A2.3.2 Hygiene and hand washing

Evidence in general population studies clearly shows a 30–40% reduction in diarrhoeal disease associated with hand washing or the proxy of presence of soap (Curtis & Cairncross, 2003; Fewtrell et al., 2005). The few studies that consider HIV-positive status indicate a protective effect of hand washing on diarrhoeal disease. Three studies were found on HIV/AIDS and hygiene. In a study on the effects of hand washing with soap on diarrhoea rates in PLHIV in the United States, Huang & Zhou (2007) found a 58% reduction in diarrhoeal incidence from 2.92 episodes of diarrhoea to 1.24 episodes. In a study of male sexual partners of Kenyan women with genital symptoms, Meier et al. (2006) found that men with reported lower hygiene behaviours were more likely to be HIV positive than the women's other sexual partners, including adjustment for confounding factors. This study used five hygiene variables, and was controlled for socioeconomic status and other potential confounders. The Lule study found that presence of soap in the household (an indicator for hand washing and general hygiene) was associated with fewer days of diarrhoea and fewer lost days of work or school due to diarrhoea. Indeed, some hygiene-related, opportunistic infections in PLHIV, such as tuberculosis or toxoplasmosis cause disease by primary infection, reinfection or recrudescence of the infectious agent (Onadeko, Joynson & Payne, 1992). In this case, it is not clear whether increased hygiene can significantly affect these diseases.

In two southern states in India, knowledge of safe water, sanitation and hygiene issues were greater among PLHIV than among the general public. Where possible, PLHIV had adopted safer water and hygiene practices, such as purifying water with some method and washing hands with soap after defecation (WSP, 2007). Research in Zambia and Malawi found that fewer than half the houses studied had a hand-washing facility and only 20% had water to use. A large gap was noted between hygiene knowledge and practice among those surveyed. Further, in Zambia, only 38% surveyed had knowledge of hygiene practices and no homes surveyed had been visited by a hygiene promoter in the previous two months.

Although solid field research provides evidence that hand washing can decrease respiratory infections in people with full immune systems (Luby et al., 2005), no similar research has been done on PLHIV. Additionally, ample evidence exists that improved body hygiene (daily bathing) and regular laundering of clothing and bed linen decrease skin infections and skin parasites (scabies, lice, bed bugs, etc.) in people with full immune systems, and is also considered to be such a basic part of human dignity that no other research is needed to justify their integration into HIV/AIDS programming.

A2.3.3 Wastewater-related risk of HIV and waterborne disease

No direct studies document HIV transmission through wastewater, but by definition, diarrhoea pathogens are waterborne. Questions have arisen about whether HIV can be transmitted through wastewater contact. As documented above, HIV is relatively unstable and even at unusually high concentrations, it loses its infectivity after a few hours, so an almost negligible risk exists for transmitting the HIV virus to household members through wastewater, especially as studies indicate that the virus is further inactivated by presence of water or urine. Studies have also shown (Ansari, Farrah & Chaudhry, 1992; Moore, 1993) that the necessary conditions for HIV transmission are absent in wastewater systems. However, pathogens causing diarrhoea remain infective and can be transmitted through wastewater, so guidelines should recommend that caregivers practice proper hygiene techniques to limit diarrhoea transmission throughout the household.

A2.4 Other programmatic evidence

A2.4.1 Cost-effectiveness

The only study on cost-effectiveness of WASH in improving PLHIV health was by Shrestha et al. (2006), separately analyzing the Lule study data. Using the programme costs from the Lule study, the researchers calculated that it cost $5.21 per diarrhoea episode averted, $0.62 per diarrhoea-day averted and $1252 per disability adjusted life year (DALY) gained. The cost per DALY was artificially high in this study for two reasons. First, the programme studied rapidly diagnosed and treated diarrhoea though mortality remained high. Second, the DALY included all programme costs, including those for start-up. If only the costs per household were calculated, it would be about $5 per year (Mermin et al., 2005) and would be comparable to the cost-effectiveness of the expanded immunization programme (tuberculosis, diphtheria, pertussis, tetanus, polio, measles) at $7 per DALY (DCP2, 2006). By comparison, the cost for ART therapy in Africa is calculated at $910 per DALY (Walensky et al., 2007).

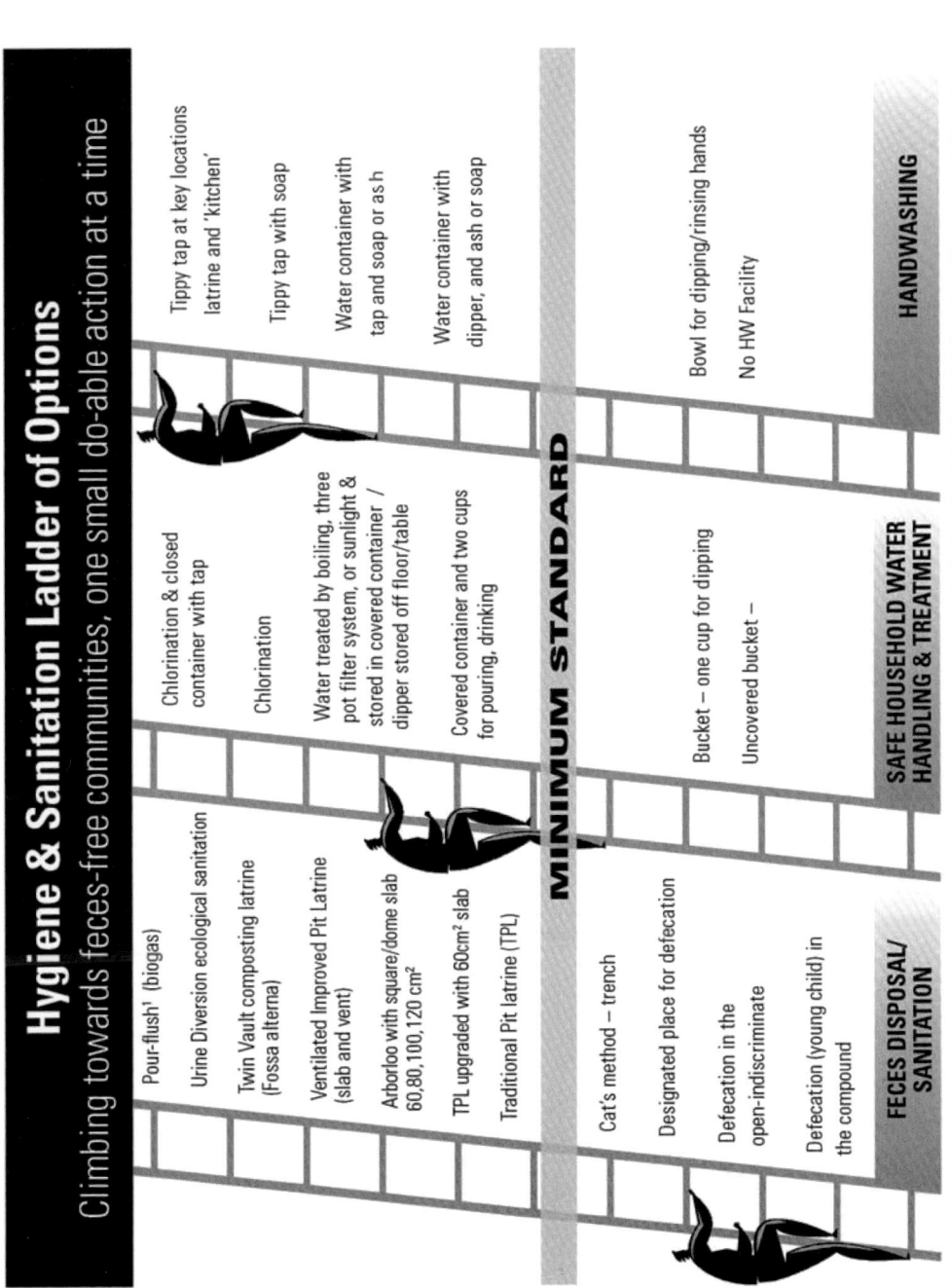

Hygiene & Sanitation Ladder of Options
Climbing towards feces-free communities, one small do-able action at a time

HANDWASHING
- Tippy tap at key locations latrine and 'kitchen'
- Tippy tap with soap
- Water container with tap and soap or ash
- Water container with dipper, and ash or soap
- Bowl for dipping/rinsing hands
- No HW Facility

SAFE HOUSEHOLD WATER HANDLING & TREATMENT
- Chlorination & closed container with tap
- Chlorination
- Water treated by boiling, three pot filter system, or sunlight & stored in covered container / dipper stored off floor/table
- Covered container and two cups for pouring, drinking
- Bucket – one cup for dipping
- Uncovered bucket –

FECES DISPOSAL/ SANITATION
- Pour-flush[1] (biogas)
- Urine Diversion ecological sanitation
- Twin Vault composting latrine (Fossa alterna)
- Ventilated Improved Pit Latrine (slab and vent)
- Arborloo with square/dome slab 60,80,100,120 cm[2]
- TPL upgraded with 60cm[2] slab
- Traditional Pit latrine (TPL)
- Cat's method – trench
- Designated place for defecation
- Defecation in the open-indiscriminate
- Defecation (young child) in the compound

MINIMUM STANDARD

Pour-flush can either be linked to septic tanks or via small bore sewerage to biogas digesters.

FAECES DISPOSAL

Counselling Card

Put the faeces of sick people, adults, children, babies, and animals in a latrine.

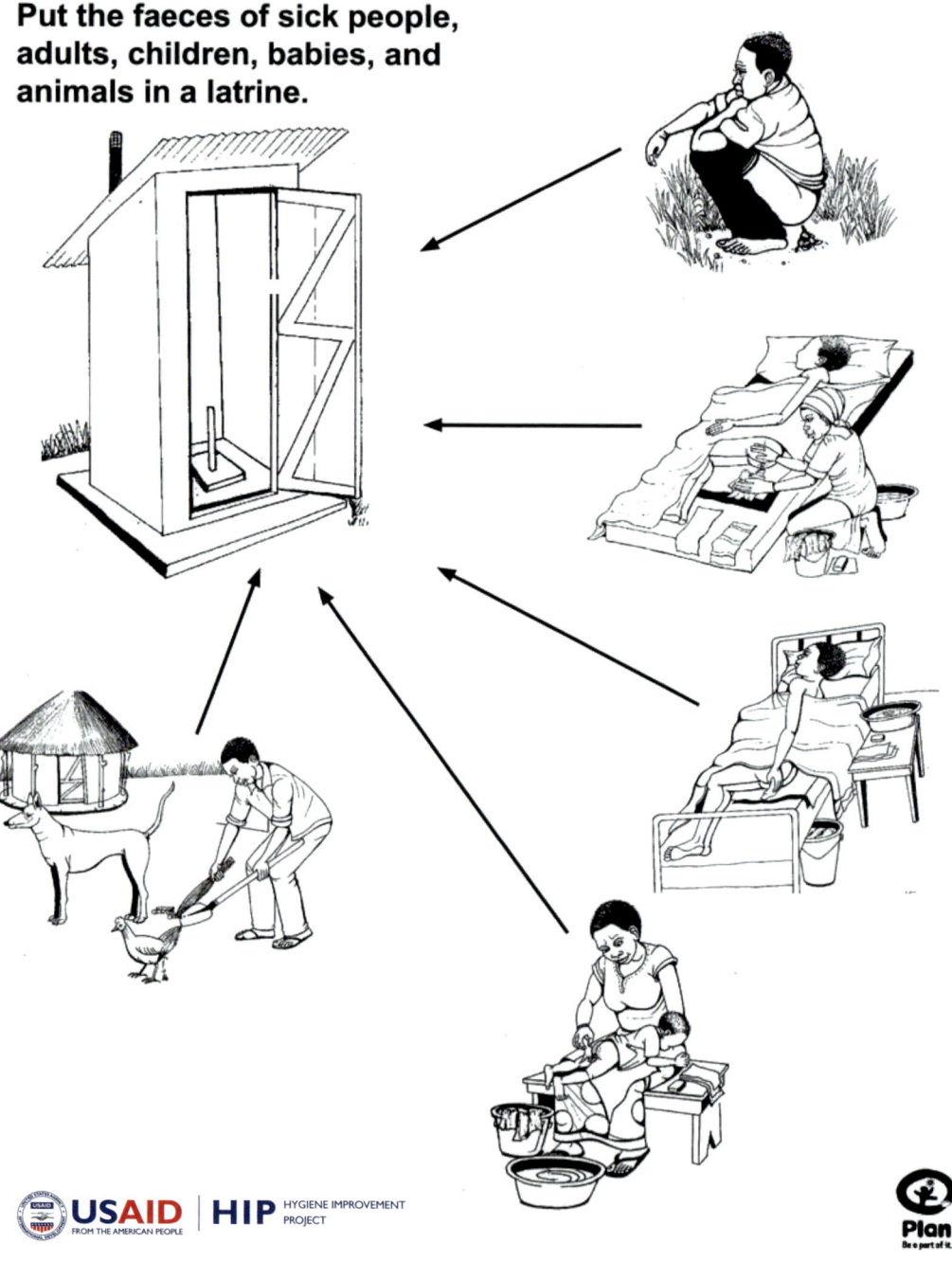

FAECES MANAGEMENT

Counselling Card

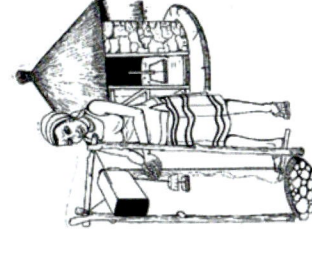

Put hand washing supplies near where sick person defecates.

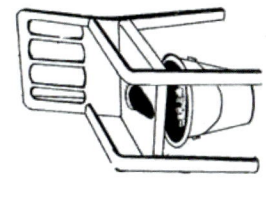

Put bucket under chair with hole in seat for indoor use.

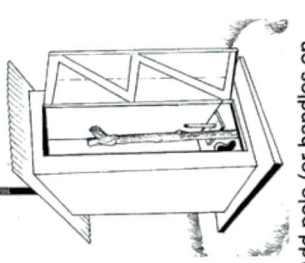

Add pole (or handles on wall) to latrine to help weak person squat or stand up.

WEAK BUT MOBILE PATIENT

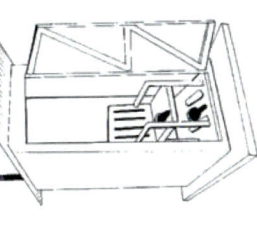

Cut hole in chair to help weak person use latrine.

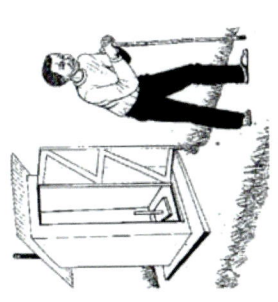

Use walking stick.

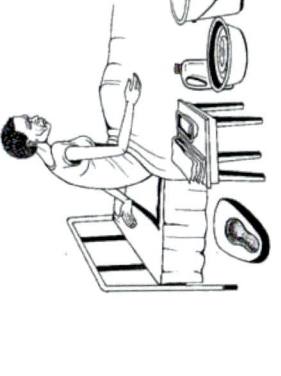

Put water, soap (or ash), and clean rags next to sick person's bed.

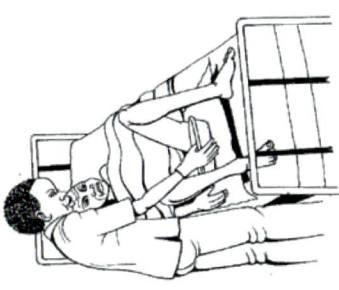

Use potty (bedpan).

BEDRIDDEN PATIENT

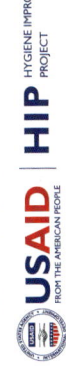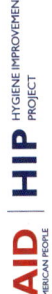

Put plastic sheet (mackintosh, kaveera) with a cloth on top under sick person's hips. Change cloth when soiled.

USAID FROM THE AMERICAN PEOPLE | HIP HYGIENE IMPROVEMENT PROJECT

Plan live as part of it

MAKING A COMMODE (POTTY CHAIR)

Counselling Card

1 Make a wooden stool or chair.

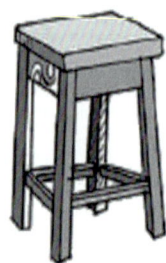

2 Cut an oval hole in the middle of the stool that "fits" the user (not too big, not too small). Smooth the edge of the hole to avoid bruising.

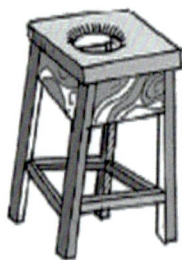

3 To use commode (potty chair):

- put a bucket beneath the hole in the stool/chair

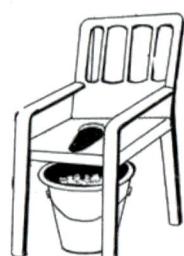

OR

- put the stool/chair over the hole in the latrine.

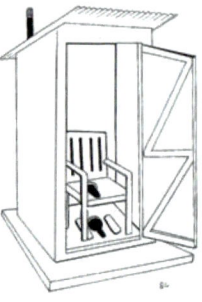

Instructions adapted from "Making Adaptations Commode/Potty Chair," Hospice Africa (Uganda).

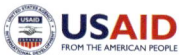 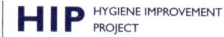

USAID FROM THE AMERICAN PEOPLE

HIP HYGIENE IMPROVEMENT PROJECT

Plan
Be a part of it.

HOW TO USE A BEDPAN

Counselling Card

1 If person can lift hips, slide the bedpan under the buttocks.

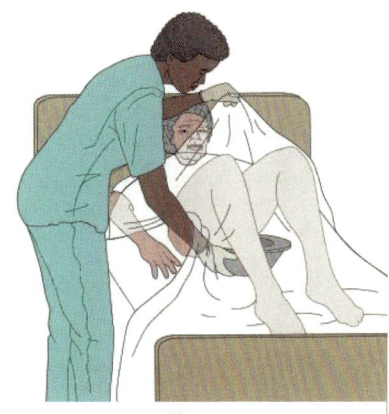

2 If person cannot lift hips:
- Turn person onto side
- Place bedpan against person's buttocks
- Assist person to roll onto bedpan

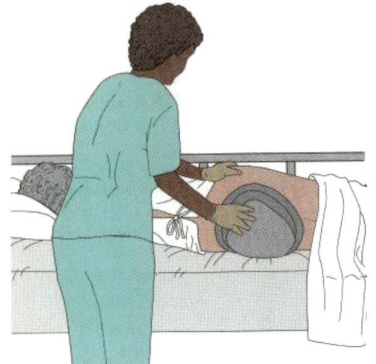

3
- After person has finished (defaecated – urinated), carefully remove bedpan without spilling
- Clean person
- Immediately put faeces – urine in latrine

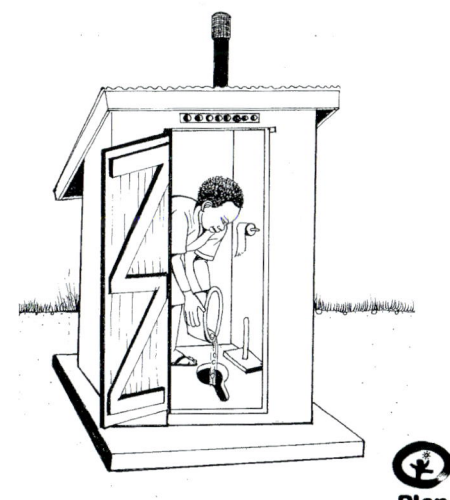

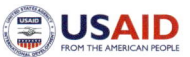 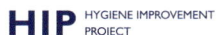

TURNING BED-BOUND CLIENT, CHANGING BED LINENS

Counselling Card

1
- Cover hands with buveera/gloves if linens are soiled.
- Bend the person's farthest arm next to his/her head and place the other arm across his/her chest.
- Cross his/her leg over the other leg.

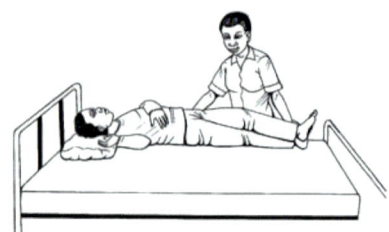

2
- Assist the person to turn to the far side of the bed.
- Place one hand on the person's shoulder and the other on his/her hip.
- Turn the person away from you onto his/her side so that they are close to the side of the bed farthest away from you.

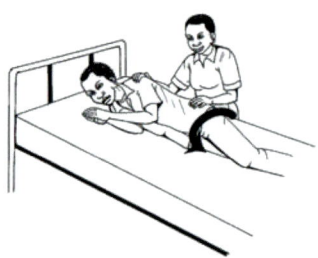

3
- On the side closest to you, loosen the bottm sheet/plastic sheet/cotton cloth.

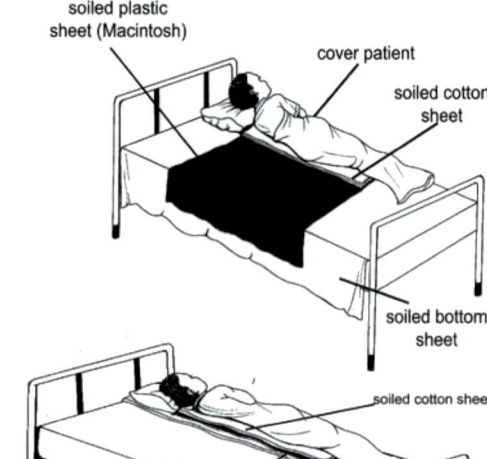

soiled plastic sheet (Macintosh)

cover patient

soiled cotton sheet

soiled bottom sheet

- Fanfold bottom linens one at a time toward the person: cotton cloth, plastic sheet, bottom sheet.
- Wipe any moisture on exposed mattress with Jik solution.

soiled cotton sheet

uncovered (bare) mattress

soiled plastic sheet (Macintosh)

soiled bottom sheet

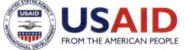 USAID FROM THE AMERICAN PEOPLE | 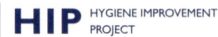 HIP HYGIENE IMPROVEMENT PROJECT

Plan
Be a part of it.

4

- Place clean bottom sheet on the exposed side of the bed by folding it lengthwise with center crease in middle of bed.
- Smooth the side nearest you and tuck the sheet under the mattress. Fanfold the top part towards the person.
- If a plastic sheet is used, repeat previous two steps with plastic sheet, placing it where the person's hips and thighs will lay.
- A plastic sheet must be completely covered with a cotton cloth. Place the the cotton cloth on top of the plastic sheet and repeat the same steps followed for the bottom and plastic sheets.

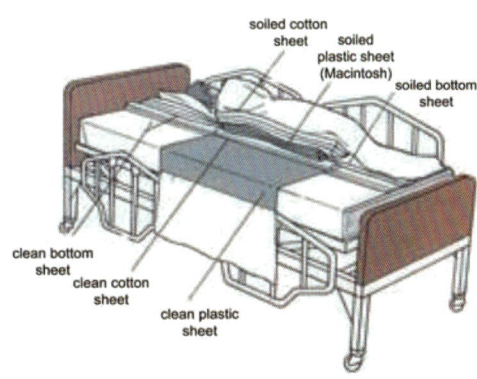

soiled cotton sheet

soiled plastic sheet (Macintosh)

soiled bottom sheet

clean bottom sheet

clean cotton sheet

clean plastic sheet

5

- Go to the other side of the bed and, repeating steps 1 and 2, position the person on the side of the bed away from you (so they are rolled onto the clean linens).
- One the side closest to you, loosen the soiled linens, if soiled, remove them one piece at a time by rolling or folding them away from you, with the side that touched the person inside the roll.
- If person is dirty , clean them, then wash gloves/buveera with soap and water (or put on clean ones).

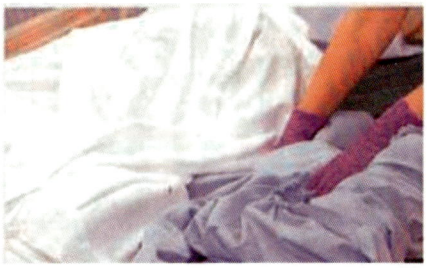

6

- Pull the clean bottom sheet, plastic sheet, and cotton cloth towards you and tuck in under matress.

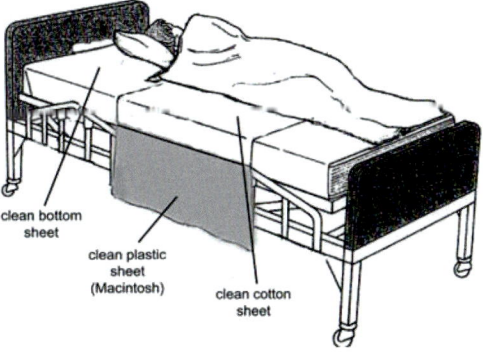

clean bottom sheet

clean plastic sheet (Macintosh)

clean cotton sheet

Tippy-Tap

A simple low-cost technology for handwashing when water is scarce

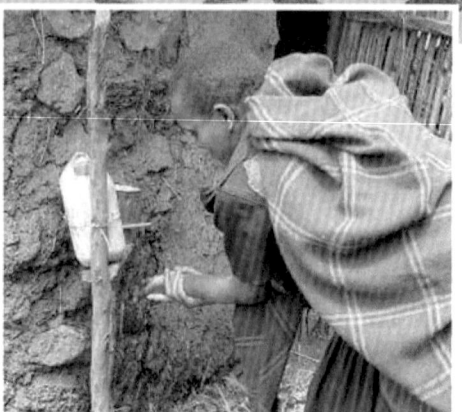

Studies have shown that proper hand-washing with soap or ash can reduce the incidence of diarrhoeal disease by 42-47 percent[1]. However, lack of access to both piped water supply and soap, is a barrier to hand washing. "Tippy Taps" are simple and economical hand-washing stations, made with commonly available materials and not dependent on a piped water supply. This publication describes how to construct and maintain a Tippy Tap.

> **TIPPY TAPS CAN BE MADE FROM A VARIETY OF LOCAL MATERIALS, INCLUDING CAST OFF PLASTIC CONTAINERS, JERRY CANS OR GOURDS. BE CREATIVE! BELOW ARE INSTRUCTIONS USING A 5 LITER JUG.**

Tippy Tap Construction

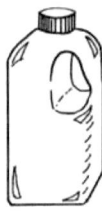

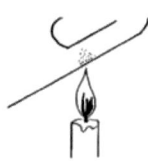

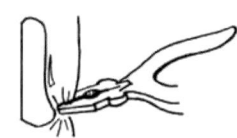

1. First, select a plastic container of approximately 5 liters, or 1.5 gallons, with a handle.

2. Then, warm the base of the handle with a candle until the plastic is soft.

3. When the base is soft, pinch the base closed with a pair of pliers and then let it cool. Make sure that no water can flow through the pinch-closed base.

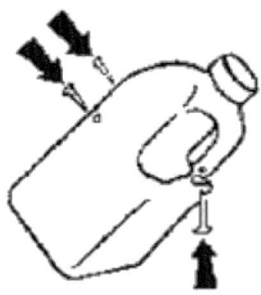

4. Heat the point of a small nail over a candle. Use the hot nail to make a small hole on the outside edge of the handle, just above the sealed area. Heat the nail again and make two larger holes on the back of the bottle. The holes should be about half way up the bottle and about a thumb-width apart. These holes will be used to thread string to hang the tippy tap. The holes need to be wide enough apart to hold the string and to be positioned so that the "full" bottle hangs at a 45 degree angle. (This picture shows a 45 degree angle.)

To Install and Use a Tippy Tap

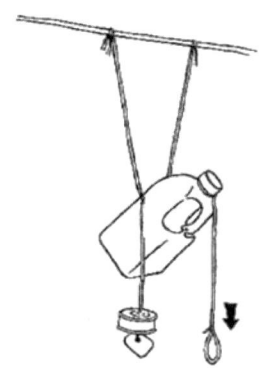

5. Hang the Tippy Tap near a latrine, kitchen, or school. Thread the string through the two holes and tie the ends of the string to a stick, a tree or stable support.

Thread a bar of soap and an empty tin can (the lid facing upwards) through another piece of string. The tin will protect the soap from rain and sun. Attach the "soap and tin" string to one of the top supporting strings. Tie a separate piece of string to the bottle cap and leave the string hanging. This string can be pulled to tip the tippy tap over for water to come out the hole in the handle.

6. Pour water into the tippy tap until the water is almost level with the holes in the back of the bottle. The tippy tap is now ready for use.

7. Use the handle or the cap to tip the container and allow water to flow out of the hole onto your hands.

Always wash with soap or ash!

Recommendations for Tippy Tap Maintenance

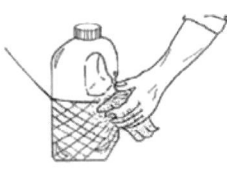

- Clean the outside of the Tippy Tap with a brush and soap daily, and clean the inside of the Tippy Tap once per week with clean water and disinfectant.

The above was adapted from the CDC website, www.cdc.gov/safewater. The original gourd tippy tap was designed by Dr. Jim Watt and Jackson Masawi at the University of Zimbabwe's rural centre. The plastic tippy tap was designed by Ralph Garnet and Dr. Jim Watt in Canada. We would like to thank CIDEPTA and PAHO for the figures and source material.

1. Curtis, Val and Sandy Cairncross (2003). "Effect of washing hands with soap on diarrhoea risk in the community, a systemic review." The Lancet: Infectious Diseases, Volume 3, May 2003.

HOW TO WASH YOUR HANDS

Counselling Card

1 Wet your hands and lather them with soap (or ash).

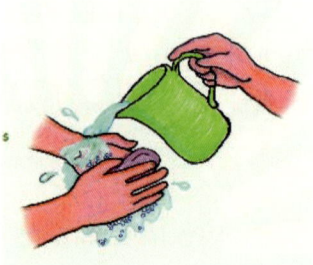

2 Rub your hands together.

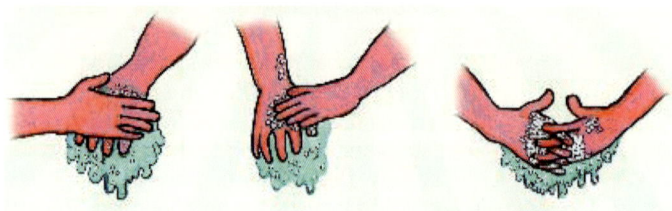

3 Rinse your hands with a stream of water.

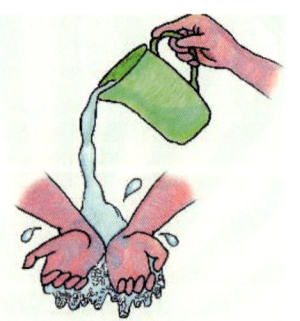

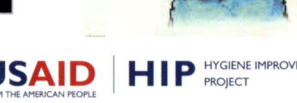

4 Shake excess water off your hands and air dry them.

USAID FROM THE AMERICAN PEOPLE | HIP HYGIENE IMPROVEMENT PROJECT

Plan Be a part of it.

MENSTRUAL PERIOD MANAGEMENT

Counselling Card

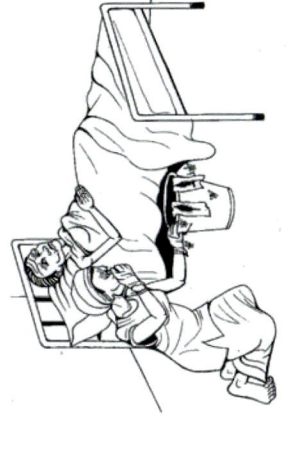

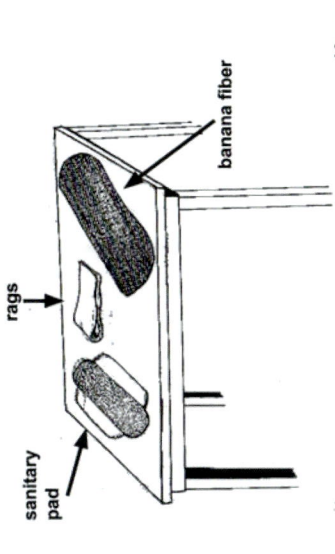

Soak up blood with sanitary pads, rags, or banana fibers.

sanitary pad

rags

banana fiber

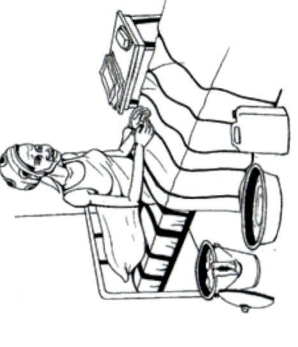

Keep clean rags, washing water, soap (or ash), and a container for soiled rags near bed-bound woman.

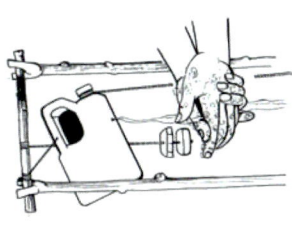

Do not store soiled rags for a long time.

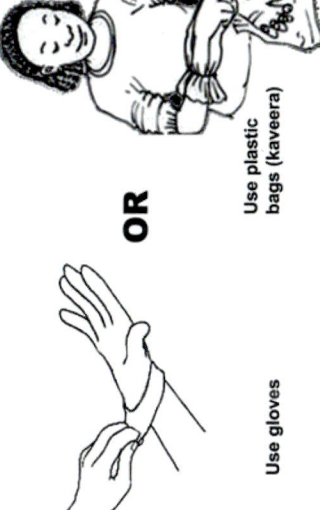

Use gloves

OR

Use plastic bags (kaveera)

Always protect hands by wearing gloves or plastic bags (kaveera) when touching someone else's blood.

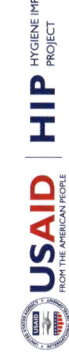

Always wash hands with soap (or ash).

USAID FROM THE AMERICAN PEOPLE

HIP HYGIENE IMPROVEMENT PROJECT

Plan Be a part of it.

Five keys to safer food

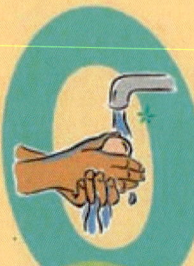

Keep clean

- Wash your hands before handling food and often during food preparation
- Wash your hands after going to the toilet
- Wash and sanitize all surfaces and equipment used for food preparation
- Protect kitchen areas and food from insects, pests and other animals

Why?

While most microorganisms do not cause disease, dangerous microorganisms are widely found in soil, water, animals and people. These microorganisms are carried on hands, wiping cloths and utensils, especially cutting boards and the slightest contact can transfer them to food and cause foodborne diseases.

Separate raw and cooked

- Separate raw meat, poultry and seafood from other foods
- Use separate equipment and utensils such as knives and cutting boards for handling raw foods
- Store food in containers to avoid contact between raw and prepared foods

Why?

Raw food, especially meat, poultry and seafood, and their juices, can contain dangerous microorganisms which may be transferred onto other foods during food preparation and storage.

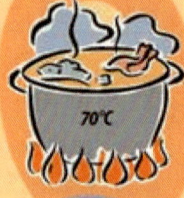

Cook thoroughly

- Cook food thoroughly, especially meat, poultry, eggs and seafood
- Bring foods like soups and stews to boiling to make sure that they have reached 70°C. For meat and poultry, make sure that juices are clear, not pink. Ideally, use a thermometer
- Reheat cooked food thoroughly

Why?

Proper cooking kills almost all dangerous microorganisms. Studies have shown that cooking food to a temperature of 70°C can help ensure it is safe for consumption. Foods that require special attention include minced meats, rolled roasts, large joints of meat and whole poultry.

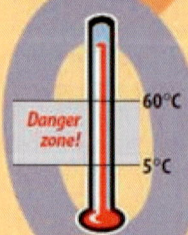

Keep food at safe temperatures

- Do not leave cooked food at room temperature for more than 2 hours
- Refrigerate promptly all cooked and perishable food (preferably below 5°C)
- Keep cooked food piping hot (more than 60°C) prior to serving
- Do not store food too long even in the refrigerator
- Do not thaw frozen food at room temperature

Why?

Microorganisms can multiply very quickly if food is stored at room temperature. By holding at temperatures below 5°C or above 60°C, the growth of microorganisms is slowed down or stopped. Some dangerous microorganisms still grow below 5°C.

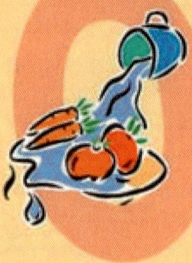

Use safe water and raw materials

- Use safe water or treat it to make it safe
- Select fresh and wholesome foods
- Choose foods processed for safety, such as pasteurized milk
- Wash fruits and vegetables, especially if eaten raw
- Do not use food beyond its expiry date

Why?

Raw materials, including water and ice, may be contaminated with dangerous microorganisms and chemicals. Toxic chemicals may be formed in damaged and mouldy foods. Care in selection of raw materials and simple measures such as washing and peeling may reduce the risk.

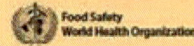
Food Safety
World Health Organization

Knowledge = Prevention

Annex 4 Things to get the community talking about and acting against stigma

Adapted from *Understanding and challenging HIV stigma: toolkit for action.*

Stigma generally arises from fear about getting HIV or AIDS and wanting to protect yourself and your family or from value-based judgements. Both can be confronted but may have slightly different solutions. In the community PLHIV and families face different forms of stigma: isolation, insults and discrimination. In some cases they are kicked out of rental accommodation or their businesses suffer because people stop buying from them.

Strategies to combat stigma are listed below.

- Involve community leaders and community-based organization in promoting anti-stigma work.

- Use PLHIV as role models and facilitators.

- Organize community meetings, peer group meetings and home visits.

- Organize drama performances.

- Make links between clinic and community.

- Inform community members what is involved in caring for PLHIV – physical care, counselling, etc.

Community meetings are important to discuss what has been learned through activities that identify stigma and to make decisions about how the community wants to solve these issues; for example, agreeing on a code of conduct, or specific support to families living with HIV and AIDS and orphans.

Make sure that people who want to make a difference are given an opportunity to state their commitment to challenge stigma publicly. Action starts with commitment and powerful commitment ensures that obstacles are challenged and overcome. The commitment of leaders serves as a role model and encouragement for others. Whenever possible, find examples of how one person's commitment led to action that made a difference in his or her community.

Different activities can get community members to identify and analyze stigma in their own community. Activities include:

- *testimonies* by PLHIV or their families about experience of living with HIV;

- *education* on facts and myths about HIV transmission;

- *language watch* – school children or youth groups make a "listening survey" to identify stigmatizing words used in the community – in media or in popular songs;

- *community mapping* of stigma of stigma points that is displayed in a prominent place in the community;

- *demonstrating positive behaviours* – community leaders demonstrate positive behaviours such as embracing PLHIV, sharing a meal and utensils, using same latrine and/or water points;

- *drama* by a youth group based on real examples – trigger for discussion;

- *pictures* drawn by youth or children – focus or starting point for discussion;

- *Training workshops* on stigma for community and peer group leaders.

A4.1 Sample activity 1: Picture-storm – a world where there is no stigma

Divide into pairs and hand out cards. Ask pairs to draw pictures and words for "a world where there is no stigma." If there is time, have them draw "before" and "after" illustrations – the world as it is – with stigma; and then as it might be – without stigma.

Discussion

Have participants explain their before and after pictures.

- What is the situation in the drawing?

- Why did they choose that particular subject/place?

- What has changed before and after? What needs to change?

- What are the obstacles to change?

- What would facilitate change?

- Who can help to facilitate change? Who is standing in the way?

- What is the first/next step in bringing about change?

- What, specifically, can we do to build this kind of world?

Post these pictures around the room to serve as inspiration for stopping stigma.

A4.2 Sample activity 2: Community group problem solving

Divide members into different groups. Have each group answer these three questions.

- What forms of stigma do you see in your community?
- What is the biggest stigma problem in your community?
- What is the source of this problem?

Have each group answer the question below.

What are some possible solutions to these problems?

As a group, identify 2–3 specific new things the community will do to stamp out stigma in this context. In addition to the community activities, ask each individual to agree to do 2–3 things on the list, so that they are involved in stopping stigma.

Be concrete, "Think big. Start small. Act now!"

A4.3 Sample activity 3: Naming stigma through key questions

Put up blank sheets of flipchart paper on different walls of the room and write a question at the top of each sheet.

- How are people living with HIV treated by the community?
- How do PLHIV feel when they are treated badly?
- How are *families* affected by HIV/AIDS?
- How are *communities* affected by HIV/AIDS?
- What are the *attitudes/feelings* of the general public toward PLHIV?
- What do people *say* about PLHIV? What WORDS do they use?
- When you come across HIV stigma, what do you *see*?
- *Why* do you think community members treat PLHIV badly?
- What are people's *fears* about HIV/AIDS?
- What are your own *fears* about working/living with PLHIV?
- What are you doing to *prevent* stigmatization toward PLHIV?
- What *messages* in the MEDIA promote stigma?

Add your own objective or topic.

Rotational brainstorming

Divide into groups and assign each group to a topic. Ask groups to brainstorm points for their topic and record them quickly. (Ask them to start writing their first thoughts immediately, not stand talking for a long time without writing.) After 3 minutes shout "CHANGE" and ask groups to move to the next topic and add points. Continue until groups have contributed ideas to all of the questions.

Rotational report back

Whole group moves around the room, looking at one topic at a time. Ask one participant to read out the points quickly and then ask for clarifications and additions. Note common or linked points.

A4.4   Sample activity 4: Mapping stigma in the community

Divide into small groups and ask each group to make a quick map of their community, showing roads and major institutions using natural objects (stones, sticks, etc). While the group makes the map on the ground, one member draws it on flipchart paper. Ask the group to indicate places where stigma occurs in the community.

Put up the maps on the front wall and make a list of places where stigma occurs.

Discussion

Who are stigmatized? Who are the stigmatizers? What forms of stigma take place in each context? How do you think people who are stigmatized would be affected?

Develop solutions for preventing or mitigating stigma in these places.

For more exercises and information on stigma related to HIV, please review the publication *Understanding and Challenging HIV Stigma: toolkit for Action,* **available** at http://www.changeproject.org **and** http://www.icrw.org.

Annex 5   Small doable actions chart

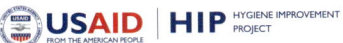

A5.1   Helping people improve their wash practices— one small doable action at a time …

① First, assess current WASH conditions of the household …

② Then negotiate a set of a few "small doable actions" that families and/or people living with HIV or AIDS are willing to try, to improve their hygiene and sanitation, and reduce diarrhoea in the home.

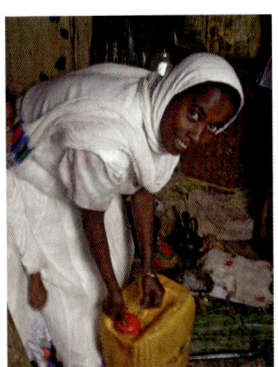

Table A5.1   Small doable actions chart

Key WASH behaviours	Assessing current conditions and practices	Negotiate a set of a few small doable actions
Water management	*Drinking water source and container* Where do people get their drinking water from? Determine/observe how people store water for drinking and the materials (jug, cup/glass) used.	Use narrow mouth ensara or 20 litre jerry can with a cover to store drinking water. Attach the cover to the ensara or jerry can using a string to keep it off the floor. Treat drinking water in the 20 litre jerry can or ensara with Wuha agar.
	Serving drinking water Watch the person provide drinking water. (Is it poured in a glass or jug? Is a dipper used? Do hands touch the water? Is the dipper kept clean and off the floor? How are the glasses stored?) – If jug is used, find out if the jug has a cover. Is there a jug for washing hands?	Pour water from jerry can or ensara into a clean cup or glass OR pour into a clean jug with cover and then pour into a clean glass. If a jug is used, the jug should have a cover and be reserved for serving drinking water only. Wash jug and its cover with soap and water every day.

Table A5.1 *continued*

Key WASH behaviours	Assessing current conditions and practices	Negotiate a set of a few small doable actions
Water management	*Keep drinking water safe and jug and glass/cup clean* Observe the practices after serving drinking water: Are the water container and jug covered? How and where is the cup/glass stored? Ask: How (with what and how often) do you clean the jug? If ensara is used to store drinking water, find out how householders clean the ensara, and how often. Explore what makes it difficult for people to store, treat, and serve drinking water safely. Find out about other existing practices related to drinking water.	Keep jerry can or ensara covered during the day and night. Put clean glass or cup upside down on a clean tray on a shelf or table. Raise storage container from floor, and store jerry can or ensara out of reach of children or animals.
Hand washing	*Find out when and how people wash their hands* Determine (ask and observe) whether soap is available, or if ash is used. Ask people to show you how they wash their hands. Determine (ask) what makes it difficult for people to wash hands with soap or ash, or/and at critical times.	Make and use tippy tap for hand washing. Place a bucket below the tippy tap to catch the water. Place the tippy tap next to the latrine, in the kitchen, and if necessary next to the bed to make it easy for PLWHA to wash, and for the caregiver to wash at critical times. *Proper hand-washing technique* Wet hands, lather with soap, ash, or sand, rub between fingers to the wrist, back of hands, fingertips, under nails. Rinse under running water. Dry in the air. Wash hands properly with water and soap or ash before meals and cooking, after using the toilet or cleaning the potty, after cleaning baby's bottom, and after attending to the patient.

Key WASH behaviours	Assessing current conditions and practices	Negotiate a set of a few small doable actions
Faeces management	*Infrastructure/equipment for proper disposal of faeces* Where do adults and children defecate? Does a latrine exist? If latrine does not exist, find out if space/land is available to construct a latrine. Is an existing latrine accessible? If latrine is available, is there a specific time where latrine is not used? What makes it difficult for people to use the latrine? Do people have a popo (plastic, clay, wooden, or old tin) that can be used? Do adults have a safe place (latrine, trash can) to dispose of faeces?	If latrine is not available, construct a latrine (ecosan latrine pit latrine or ventilated improved pit latrine) with superstructure (walls) from local materials. Use latrine and/or the potty and/or plastic bag for all family members. Put a handful of ash in the latrine after defecation (to get rid of the smell and the flies). Put ash/sand in popo before use. Immediately dispose of the faeces in the latrine or trash can. Put used paper in a tin.
	After defecation Ask: What do you do after you defecate? (Probe after using popo or latrine)	Wash popo with water and soap, ash or sand. Place potty out of the reach of children Wash hands with water and soap or ash after disposing of the faeces from the potty or cleaning a baby's or anyone's bottom, or when attending to a patient.

Table A5.1 *continued*

Key WASH behaviours	Assessing current conditions and practices	Negotiate a set of a few small doable actions
Diarrhoea management for bed-bound PLWHA	*Sleeping pattern/practices of bedridden PLWHA* Observe type of bed, mat or mattress. Is the bed mat or mattress covered with bed sheets? Is the bed, mat or mattress covered with plastic? Is the plastic covered with a bed sheet or piece of cloth?	Caregiver should spread a plastic sheet (or some opened out plastic bags) across the part of the bed under the buttocks and completely cover the plastic with a piece of cloth. (Have several pieces of cloth available for use so when one is soiled it can be immediately replaced with another. These can be made from old skirts, dresses, bed sheets.)
	Care for bed bound PLWHA suffering from diarrhoea How does a caregiver take care of a bedridden person during diarrhoea? How do caregivers clean up diarrhoea? From body, from sheets, from bed?	Caregivers should use gloves when caring for PLWHA suffering from diarrhoea. Caregivers should wash faeces-stained/soiled bed sheet and cloth of the sick person with water and soap and dry it in the sun. Caregivers should always wash hands with water and soap before and after caring for PLWHA suffering from diarrhoea.
	PLWHA is alone If a caregiver is not available, what does a bedridden person do after having diarrhoea?	If PLWHA is alone and very weak in bed, after defecating, roll over and reposition; lean on the side while waiting for someone to help.
Menstruation management for PLWHA	*Protection during menstruation* Find out what material (piece of cloth, pad, others …) is used for protection during menstruation.	Use clean a piece of cloth from linen or cotton material or a clean pad. Store the used piece of cloth in a plastic bag during daytime to prevent the contact with the blood-stained material.

Table A5.1 *continued*

Key WASH behaviours	Assessing current conditions and practices	Negotiate a set of a few small doable actions
Menstruation management for PLWHA	*Hygiene during menstruation* Where do you dispose of the blood-stained material (piece of cloth, pad ...)? If it is washed, ask: how do you wash it? How (when and where) do you dry it?	Dispose of the used pad in the latrine or in the trash can. *Washing the cloth* Wash the used piece of cloth with soap and water at night. (Caregivers should wear gloves to protect their hands.) Dry on the line/hang at night and collect early in the morning. Keep the clean and dry pieces of cloth in a clean box after menstruation.
	Cleaning the stained dress/bed sheet What do you do with the stained cloth/dress? What do you do with the stained bed sheet?	Remove the dress, linen/bed sheet and wash with soap and water. Dry the dress, bed sheet/linen outside the house under the sun.

Annex 6 Competencies of home-based care workers in hygiene at household level

Hygiene at household level refers to water, faeces and diarrhoea management as well as hand washing, and safe handling of menstrual blood.

A home-based care worker should be able to:

- assess *current level* of household hygiene in regard to

    - personal hygiene of household members – hand washing;

    - soap availability and use for hand washing;

    - alternative to soap such as ash and sand;

    - timing for washing hands;

    - water storage, use, and safety;

    - faeces disposal;

    - latrine availability;

    - alternative to latrine where latrine is not available;

    - care of sick householders and bedbound members – diarrhoea management;

    - safe disposal of blood stained clothes/materials (in menstruating women)

- assess hygiene *needs* of households in regard to

    - personal hygiene of household members – hand washing (soap availability and use for hand washing, alternative to soap such as ash and sand, timing for washing hands);

    - water storage, use, and safety;

    - faeces disposal (latrine availability, alternative to latrine where latrine is not available, care of sick householders and bedbound members – diarrhoea management, safe disposal of blood-stained clothes/materials [in menstruating women]);

- communicate effectively and respectfully with household members on

    - current hygiene practices;

    - maintaining good hygiene practices that are being implemented;

    - identifying certain practice(s) that need changing;

- alternative improved practice(s) (presenting and discussing small doable actions to improve the practice(s));

- feasible alternative practice(s);

- changing household behaviour(s) and practice(s);

- reinforcing and solving problems around new behaviours – helping household members overcome difficulties encountered in adopting a new set of small doable actions

- demonstrate

  - hand washing – with soap and water;

  - hand washing with ash/sand;

  - how to make a tippy tap and maintain a clean tippy tap;

  - safe drinking water storage and treatment;

  - how to keep drinking water safe using local materials to provide safe water storage containers/lids and keeping water away from children and animals;

  - alternatives to latrines (e.g. bedpan where no latrine is available);

  - how to improve privacy for all household members (including sick members) when using latrine/bedpan;

  - use of local materials to make bedpan for bedbound person;

  - how to care for a bedbound person with diarrhoea;

  - how to care for bedbound women who have blood-stained clothes;

  - how to collect and report on progress in integrating WASH care at household level

- provide support, guidance, and follow-up for households implementing small doable actions.

Glossary

Acquired immunodeficiency syndrome (AIDS)	Morbidity resulting from infection with the human immunodeficiency virus.
Antiretroviral medicines	Medications to treat infection with retroviruses, such as HIV.
Condominial latrines	Latrines used by residents of a housing block.
Disinfection	Killing of infectious agents outside the body by direct exposure to chemical or physical agents. Disinfection is necessary only for diseases spread by indirect contact.
Flocculant	A chemical that encourages flocculation, which is the process where particles that are suspended in a liquid come out of suspension and clump together.
Guidelines	Guidelines aim to streamline particular processes according to a set routine. By definition, guidelines are not mandatory (whereas protocols generally are mandatory). Guidelines are issued or adopted by an organization (governmental or private) to make the actions of its employees more predictable, and presumably of higher quality.
Handbooks	Handbooks provide information to supplement guidelines; they specify processes further, and often include job aids or counselling tools to ensure that processes are implemented properly.
Hand washing	Washing hands with soap and water, and drying thoroughly.
Human excreta	Includes faeces, urine, menstrual blood, sputum and sweat.
Human immunodeficiency virus (HIV)	A virus mainly transmitted during sexual intercourse or through exposure to blood or blood products. HIV causes acquired immunodeficiency syndrome (AIDS).
Latrines	Simple, shared toilets.

Negotiating improved practice	Working with individuals to solve problems and remove barriers to behaviour change.
Opportunistic infections	Infections that are common in people with compromised immune systems.
Pit latrine	Simple and cheaper latrines, usually a hole in the ground possibly with a floor plate.
Policies	Policies are generally national or regional documents that state a set of basic principles and associated guidelines that were formulated and are enforced by the governing body. Their purpose is to influence and determine decisions, actions and other matters.
Potable water	Water of sufficient quality for drinking without risk of harm.
Rolling boil	Boiling to the point where large bubbles begin to come to the surface.
Sanitation	Safe handling and disposal of human excreta (faeces, urine, menstrual blood, sputum and sweat), management of wastes (including trash, wastewater, storm water, sewage and hazardous wastes) and control of disease vectors (such as mosquitoes and flies).
Slow sand filter	Filters that use biological processes to clean water, including filtration through fine sand and the biological activity of bacteria, fungi and other aquatic organisms.
Standards	Technical specifications or procedures that lay out characteristics of a product or procedure (e.g. levels of quality, performance, safety or dimensions).
Tippy tap	A simple system for washing hands with very little water consisting of a plastic jug, gourd or local receptacle with a tap or opening, which can be tipped without using the hands.
Turbidity	The cloudiness of a fluid caused by suspended solids. Turbidity can be measured in nephelometric yurbidity units (NTU) using a nephelometer, which detects how light is scattered by the suspended particles.

Universal precautions	Using protective barriers (e.g. gloves, gowns, masks or protective eyewear) to reduce a caregiver's risk of exposure to materials potentially infected with HIV or other bloodborne pathogens.
Vectors	Organisms that transmit pathogens from humans to humans or from animal hosts to humans.